# FEATURES

WINTER 2021 • NUMBER 26

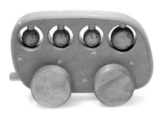
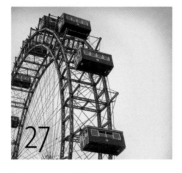
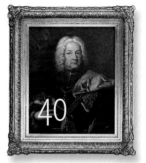
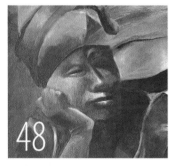
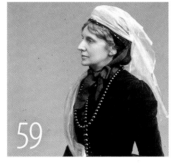
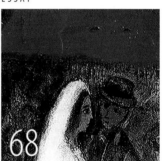
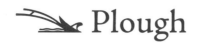
Plough

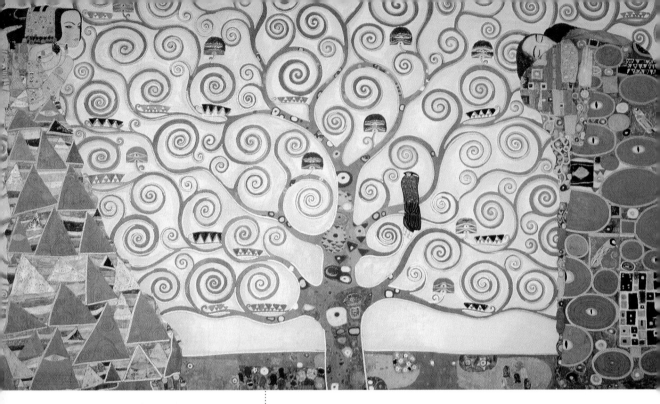

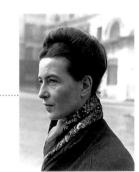

# DEPARTMENTS

# WEB EXCLUSIVES

plough.com/web26

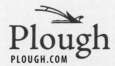

# Plough
**PLOUGH.COM**

**EDITOR:** Peter Mommsen
**SENIOR EDITORS:** Maureen Swinger, Sam Hine, Susannah Black
**EDITOR-AT-LARGE:** Caitrin Keiper
**MANAGING EDITOR:** Shana Goodwin
**POETRY EDITOR:** A. M. Juster
**DESIGNERS:** Rosalind Stevenson, Miriam Burleson
**CREATIVE DIRECTOR:** Clare Stober
**COPY EDITORS:** Wilma Mommsen, Priscilla Jensen
**FACT CHECKER:** Suzanne Quinta
**MARKETING DIRECTOR:** Trevor Wiser
**INTERNATIONAL EDITIONS:** Ian Barth (UK), Kim Comer (German),
Chungyon Won (Korean), Allen Page (French)
**FOUNDING EDITOR:** Eberhard Arnold (1883–1935)

Plough Quarterly No. 26: What Are Families For?
Published by Plough Publishing House, ISBN 978-1-63608-014-7
Copyright © 2021 by Plough Publishing House. All rights reserved.

**EDITORIAL OFFICE**
151 Bowne Drive
Walden, NY 12586
T: 845.572.3455
info@plough.com

United Kingdom
Brightling Road
Robertsbridge
TN32 5DR
T: +44(0)1580.883.344

**SUBSCRIBER SERVICES**
PO Box 8542
Big Sandy, TX 75755
T: 800.521.8011
subscriptions@plough.com

Australia
4188 Gwydir Highway
Elsmore, NSW
2360 Australia
T: +61(0)2.6723.2213

Plough Quarterly (ISSN 2372-2584) is published quarterly by
Plough Publishing House, PO Box 398, Walden, NY 12586.
Individual subscription $32 / £24 / €28 per year.
Subscribers outside the United Kingdom and European Union pay in US dollars.
Periodicals postage paid at Walden, NY 12586 and at additional mailing offices.
POSTMASTER: Send address changes to
Plough Quarterly, PO Box 8542, Big Sandy, TX 75755.

Front cover: artwork by Yulia Brodskaya, 2020; used with permission;
*artyulia.co.uk*. Inside front cover: artwork by Catherine Panebianco, 2019; used
with permission; *catherinepanebianco.com*. Back cover: artwork by Carolyn Olson,
2020; used by permission; *carolynolson.net*.

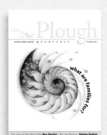

**ABOUT THE COVER:**
In the cover artwork *Shell Spiral* by Yulia
Brodskaya, circles of many patterns and sizes are
grouped together, just as individual families are
connected via kinship and community. No one
stands alone, as cells of fellowship include others
who would otherwise be isolated — the single, the
elderly, lonely neighbors. The offshoots suggest
the budding next generation as new families are
formed, and the spiral toward the center of origin
points us to our ancestors.

# FAMILY & FRIENDS

## AROUND THE WORLD

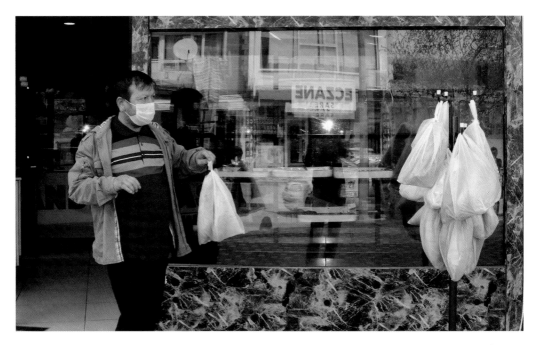

## Askıda Ekmek: Is There Bread on the Hook?

### Metin Erdem

Bread for the poor is hung outside a bakery in Turkey.

There is a bakery near our apartment in Maltepe, Istanbul, that makes more than fifteen hundred breads, biscuits, pastries, and cakes every day. You can smell the fresh bread calling you from hundreds of feet away.

One recent morning at the bakery I saw a sign, "Askıda Ekmek 37," which means there are now thirty-seven loaves of "bread on the hook" – free for anybody in need. People come and ask, *"Askıda ekmek var mi?"* "Is there bread on the hook?" and if they can't pay, they can take a loaf of bread for free. The baker told me that almost one hundred loaves are given every day. At times a customer pays for two loaves but only takes one, and the other is hung on the hook.

The tradition of "Askıda Ekmek" can be traced to the Ottoman Empire, which had the principle, "Let the people live and so the state will live." With Islam as the dominant religion, people recognize Muhammad's instruction: "He who sleeps contentedly while his neighbors sleep hungry did not believe in my message." Still today hospitality is very important in Turkish culture, especially in the villages. People believe that you are a guest of God and they will invite you in to share their food and home.

## The Breaking Ground Project

### Susannah Black

"It's April 2020," we *Plough* editors thought to ourselves a few months ago. "Why not spice up our apocalypse by partnering with a bunch of Canadians and Reformed folks in starting a new

online magazine?" This may seem like an odd choice, but we're very pleased with how it's worked out.

*Breaking Ground* is a new media project of the Canadian think tank Cardus, run in partnership with Cardus's magazine *Comment*, The Davenant Institute, and other Christian organizations. Spearheaded by *Comment* editor-in-chief Anne Snyder, the project has as its senior editor *Plough's* Susannah Black; many others in the *Plough* orbit are also involved.

This year has thrown challenge after challenge in our faces. We need, on an emergency basis, to be wise. *Breaking Ground* is dedicated to marshaling the wisdom of the Christian traditions – from Anabaptist, to Reformed, to Catholic – to face the current crisis head-on.

With podcasts, videos, and a series of live events, as well as essays from those whose voices – familiar and unfamiliar – need to be heard, *Breaking Ground* is doing just what we hoped it would: it's building community, building connections, and providing an outlet for some of the most interesting and useful writing that 2020 has produced, guided by two thousand years of Christian social thought. We're so glad to be fellow travelers on their voyage.

*breakingground.us*

## Special Announcement: Rhina Espaillat Poetry Award

In summer 2021, *Plough* will announce the winners of its first annual Rhina Espaillat Poetry Award. The winning poet will receive a two thousand dollar award and the winning poem will be published in *Plough*. In addition, two finalists will receive two hundred and fifty dollars as

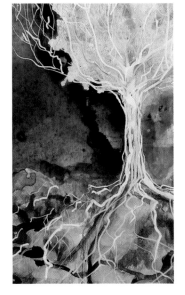

well as publication in *Plough*.

This award honors the achievements of the great Dominican-American poet, translator, and public school teacher Rhina Polonia Espaillat. The Rhina

Espaillat Poetry Award will be awarded for an original poem of not more than fifty lines that reflects her lyricism, empathy, and ability to find grace in everyday events of life.

In contrast to most other poetry competitions, *Plough* will not contract out judging of this award to a prominent poet. Instead, *Plough*'s new poetry editor A. M. Juster will select approximately twenty poems for further consideration, and then the editors will reach a consensus on the winner and the two finalists.

Submissions will open in early 2021, and the deadline for submissions is March 30, 2021. All poems must be submitted electronically via the contest webpage. All decisions of the editors will be final. Results will be announced in early summer at *Plough.com,* and by email to all contestants. For details, visit *plough.com/poetryaward.*

Petra Zantingh, *Choosing Life Tree* (detail).

Rhina Espaillat

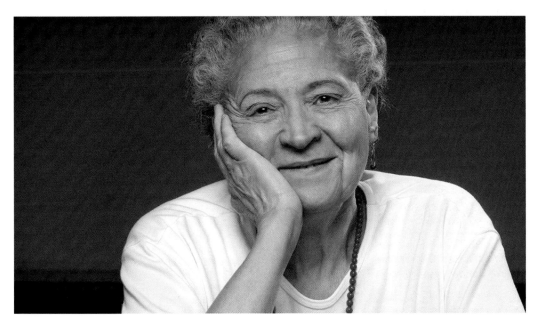

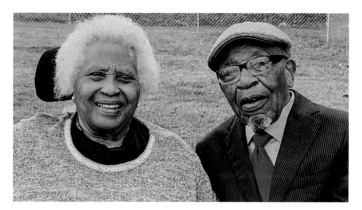

## Zoom Bible Study with Dr. John M. Perkins

### David Burleson

Dr. John M. Perkins is known for many things: his work in racial reconciliation; Christian community development; his books on justice, faith, and race. He has served as an adviser to presidents and a neighbor to gang leaders. He and his wife, Vera Mae, have just celebrated their seventieth wedding anniversary (he is ninety and she is eighty-seven). But his greatest love and passion is teaching the Bible.

I met John in 1984 when I went to Pasadena to visit a childhood friend who was volunteering with him for the summer. John convinced me to stay, and for three years we worked together building up his ministry to the children of the drug dealers and prostitutes in the neighborhood. But on Tuesday mornings at 5:30 a.m. we had Bible study – mostly the First Letter of John, but also John's Gospel.

When Covid-19 forced everyone into an unnatural isolation, I spoke with John about participating in his Bible study using Zoom. Over the past months,

these gatherings have grown and have become a focal point for what is affecting Christians around the country. John has invited many different speakers and teachers to join him.

John's Bible studies are challenging; the gospel message is so simple, yet so demanding. As he reminds us over and over, God's longing is that we might know him, be known by him, and make him known to all people. That is the good news. Learn more or join the Bible studies here: *jvmpf.org/drperkinsbiblestudy*.

## Poet in This Issue

Rachel Hadas studied classics at Harvard, poetry at Johns Hopkins, and comparative literature at Princeton. Since 1981 she has taught in the English Department at Rutgers University, and has also taught courses in literature and writing at Columbia and Princeton. She is the author of many books of poetry, prose, and translations, including *Poems for Camilla* (Measure Press, 2018).

Read her poems "Trying to Get to School" and "Lyric Leap" on page 38. ⟶

**STATEMENT OF OWNERSHIP, MANAGEMENT, AND CIRCULATION**

**(Required by 39 U.S.C. 3685)**

1. Title of publication: Plough Quarterly. 2. Publication No: 0001-6584. 3. Date of filing: October 1, 2020. 4. Frequency of issue: Quarterly. 5. Number of issues published annually: 4. 6. Annual subscription price: $32.00. 7. Complete mailing address of known office of publication: Plough Quarterly, P.O. Box 398, Walden, NY 12586. 8. Same. 9. Publisher: Plough Publishing House, same address. Editor: Peter Mommsen, same address. Managing Editor: Sam Hine, same address. 10. Owner: Plough Publishing House, P.o. Box 398, Walden, NY 12586. 11. Known bondholders, mortgages, and other securities: None. 12. The purpose, function, and nonprofit status of this organization and the exempt status for federal income tax purposes have not changed during preceding 12 months. 13. Publication Title: Plough Quarterly. 14. Issue date for circulation data below: September 1, 2020. 15. Extent and nature of circulation: Average No. copies of each issue during preceding 12 months: A. Total number of copies (net press run)—12,625. B.1. Mailed outside-county paid subscriptions: 8,513. B.2. Mailed in-county paid subscriptions: 0. B.3. Paid distribution outside the mails including sales through dealers and carriers, street vendors, counter sales, and other non-USPS paid distribution: 0. B.4. Other classes mailed through the USPS: 0. C. Total paid distribution: 8,513. D.1. Free distribution by mail: Outside-county—1,452. D.2. In-county—0. D.3. Other classes mailed through the USPS—0. Free distribution outside the mail—0. E. Total free distribution: 1,452. F. Total Distribution: 9,965. G. Copies not distributed: 2,660. H. Total: 12,625. I. Percent paid—85.43%. Actual No. copies of single issue published nearest to filing date: A. 13,000. B.1. 9,615. B.2. 0. B.3. 0. B.4. 0. C. 9,615. D.1. 1,304. D.2. 0. D.3. 0. D.4. 0. E. 1,304. F. 10,919. G. 2,081. H. 13,000. I. 88.06%. Electronic copy circulation: Average No. copies of each issue during preceding 12 months: A. Total No. Electronic Copies: 208. B. Total paid print copies plus paid electronic copies: 8,721. C. Total print distribution plus paid electronic copies: 10,173. D. Percent paid: 85.73%. Actual No. copies of single issue published nearest to filing date: A. 236. B. 9,851. C. 11,155. D. 88.31%. 17. Publication of Statement of Ownership: Winter 2021. 18. I certify that the statements made by me above are correct and complete. Sam Hine, Editor, September 30, 2020. ⟶

# FORUM ≈
## LETTERS FROM READERS

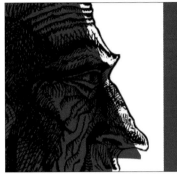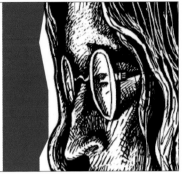

**BUT FIRST** . . . a note from the editors. Beginning in our next issue, our "Forum" section will become a place for a more curated conversation about the subjects raised by our authors. Taking our inspiration from the golden age of blogging, we'll be soliciting responses from a variety of people – and accepting unsolicited contributions as well. We'll be looking for in-depth engagement and lively back-and-forth. So give it a shot – agree, disagree, tell us why, give us stories and examples. Contributions may be edited for length and clarity, and may be published in any medium. Please include your name and the city or town you're writing from. Send contributions to *letters@plough.com*.

## Progress and Presumption

*On Natalia Osipova and Elena Avinova's adaptation of Dostoyevsky's "The Grand Inquisitor" in "Regeneration," Plough's special 2020 digital issue:* I cannot tell you how much I look forward to receiving my *Plough* issue. Sitting down and reading the essays, enjoying the art, just having it in my hands serves as an oasis of sanity and tranquility.

The graphic novel of "The Grand Inquisitor" episode in *The Brothers Karamazov* was very well timed – I will buy a few copies for those who lack the wisdom to subscribe.

As I grow older, I too think there has to be a better way; I pray that God will reveal a path. Paul Kingsnorth has noted: "One of the dangerous things about the story of progress is that we don't think it's a story. We think it's the truth." We cannot deny the advances made over

the centuries – I, for one, welcome the advances in dentistry. The more you think about progress, the more you realize that it is simply intimacy with tools and technology. But the more technologically advanced we become, the more dependent we become on tools: tools that now control us in the sense that we have freely given them control over various aspects of our lives. Once control has been surrendered, it is challenging to regain – requiring a tech detox that rarely lasts.

Simply, thank you for *Plough*. I look forward to every issue and am grateful to have discovered your publication. It helps me find calm and quiet in an otherwise messy and noisy life.

*Jean-Philippe Peltier, Monument, Colorado*

## Madonna House Greetings

*On the Autumn 2020 issue, "Solidarity":* I was delighted to get two hard copies of the Autumn issue of *Plough* in the mail yesterday. I have been reading things online, but it doesn't replace the "wholistic" experience of the issue in your hands. One of the priests has

been joking with me when he sees me at the computer not typing, "You're not reading *Plough* again?!"

So far no Covid cases within our Madonna House community. We're being prudent about our activities away from the community, and we're doing well. We have been able to receive new guests, which has been a blessing (of course, they go through testing before they enter). But as hospitality is one of the most important things we offer, it has been good to have been able to practice it concretely again.

I've just read Peter Mommsen's book *Homage to a Broken Man*. What an incredible person J. Heinrich Arnold was: "I would rather trust and be betrayed thousands of times than mistrust for a single day." Our foundress Catherine Doherty liked to say: "Trust the untrustworthy" – a call to Gospel living. She had another line: "Pain is the kiss of Christ." I think Arnold understood that one well too.

We pray that you are well. We're in the midst of harvest and the Lord has indeed been generous this year – an abundance in almost all the crops. We were able to

From Elena Avinova, *The Grand Inquisitor* (Plough, 2020)

give away three truckloads of squash. We killed our chickens earlier in the week and will all go together to begin to harvest the potatoes in a couple of days. Being all together doing a job is good for unity and family life.

*Teresa Gehred, Madonna House,*
*Combermere, Ontario, Canada*

## Arc of Justice

*On Eugene F. Rivers's and Jacqueline C. Rivers's "Black Lives Matter and the Church," Autumn 2020:* What a refreshing commentary on where we are as a nation. Rev. and Dr. Rivers have brought such light of understanding to a complex issue. Most of all, I agree with their idea that this is the moment of the intercessors: those who've been called to pray and will not stop praying until something happens. It's Joel 2:13 time: time to tear our hearts and not the outer garments of our past. As the church, we must take a true stand, repent from the inside of our hearts, then repent for the error of our ways where we have not addressed these issues of racism. And then it'll be Joel 2:14 time: "Who knows what the Lord will do?" Let's continue to have intelligent conversations like these, that let us remember that the wheat and the tares grow together now, and God said he'll do the separating when he comes.

*Gerald L. Johnson, Corona, California*

## Political Appetites

*On John D. Roth's "The Anabaptist Vision of Politics," Spring 2020:* I'll echo Roth's central point: we must not be in thrall to a nation or government. We are not to think that real power lies in Washington, he writes. Of course, realistically, unimaginable amounts of tangible power lie there. It's this that we can easily find ourselves in thrall to: that a nation has "a sacred right to –", "a sacred duty to –", that it is "a beacon of –", and so on. Even "That's not who we are" has this flavor of the sacred. . . .

The political is such a dangerous thing because it's an animal with its eyes in its stomach: it has to devour a thing before it can see if it's real. We can't see anything – a doctor, a public works project, a school, an art form, God, Allah, without knowing its political standing. There's always the question: "Is your church liberal? Is it conservative? Is it progressive?" There is a refusal to even attempt to see things in the light of the non-political, to not give everything to Caesar. We must, however, make that attempt.

*Dan Ryan, Philadelphia, Pennsylvania*

## The Vital Promise of Christian Education

*On Richard Hughes Gibson's "The Cassiodorus Necessity," Plough.com:* As a Wheaton graduate, I appreciate your deeply historical and detailed argument for the "Cassiodorus Necessity." My wife and I are neck-deep in establishing twenty Christian schools in Spain over the next twenty years. We subscribe to the Cassiodorus Necessity and believe that the work ethic, moral beauty, and "loving God with all our minds" of the Christian intellectual tradition are vital to raising a generation of leaders in Spain. (We desperately need philanthropists who are driven by this necessity to invest!) Thank you for your stimulating essay.

*Timothy Westergren, Madrid, Spain*

## Pain Shared, Pain Relieved

*On Kurt Armstrong's "My Mean Brain," Plough.com:* Your article means the world to me – I thought I was the only one. We probably have theological differences but this article overpowers any of them in its richness and insightfulness. Hang on and never quit – this article is proof that you are an effective minister and top-notch writer. He who began the good work that is in you will be faithful to bring it to abundant harvest.

*Shelly Jordan, Waterloo, Ontario*

You must be reading my mind! I too live with a mood disorder and battle regularly with these kinds of thoughts. This is a really encouraging piece and it always helps to know that one is not alone in the struggle. Thank you for sharing your experience. I think I'm going to make my own "GO TO HELL" card!

*Tim O'Regan, Brisbane, Australia*

## Concise and Gratifying Feedback

*On Phil Christman's "The Future's Back: Time Loops in Rick Perlstein's Reaganland, Louise Erdrich's The Night Watchman, and Erica Hunt's Jump the Clock," Plough.com:*

This might just be the best essay I've read about my book.

*Rick Perlstein, Chicago, Illinois*

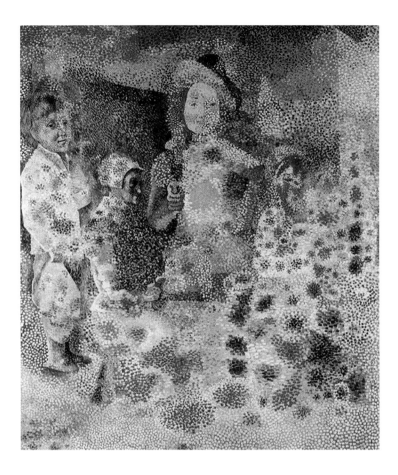

# Family Matters

PETER MOMMSEN

THERE IS A STORY about the modern family and it goes like this: Families are in crisis, and the cause is moral breakdown. Our society raises ever fewer of its young in two-parent homes; people are getting married ever later (if at all), long past their prime child-bearing years; in fact, swelling cohorts of the young are uninterested in any committed relationship – or even in sex. To be sure, members of the educated classes, if they marry, still practice fairly traditional family values (even if they don't preach them). But among the rest of the population, a pattern of family instability marked by serial cohabitation and fatherless homes swamps any positive trends. And even the stably married are, as a group, complicit in cratering birthrates, which are bound to cause grave economic and social ills as the old come to outnumber the young. We urgently need a deep renewal of our family culture, supported by public policies that strengthen traditional marriage and encourage childbearing.

Pablo Picasso, *The Happy Family* (Le Retour du baptême, d'après Le Nain), 1917

This is the narrative that social conservatives have been telling in various versions since at least 1966, when the phrase "family values" was invented. Of course, theirs isn't the only story out there. Here's another: Families are in crisis, and the cause is neoliberal capitalism. Our economic system undermines people's ability to form and sustain healthy families in a host of ways: the job market demands geographic mobility, scattering extended families and dividing generations; employment pressures make a regular home life impossible for many parents; too many children attend public schools doomed to inequality because of residential segregation by class and race. Meanwhile, our prison system deprives millions of children of their fathers and mothers – in the United States, five million children under fourteen have a parent who at some point in their lives has been incarcerated. We need structural changes in society so that all families can flourish: parental leave, guaranteed healthcare, flexible work hours for parents, zoning reform, restorative justice.

> The biological family, evidently, matters greatly; but in the order of our loves, it should come a distinct second.

These two stories, despite being associated with opposite sides of the partisan divide, don't exclude each other; both are, I believe, in large part true. But both tend to glide past the need to reckon with a more fundamental question: What are families, and what are they for?

One reason not to assume we already know the answer is the word *family* itself. As progressives are fond of pointing out, its meaning is historically slippery (though not necessarily in the ways we moderns would prefer). The English word derives from the Latin *familia,* which referred to an entire multigenerational household under one male head, including its servants and freedmen – and which, jarringly, doesn't originally refer to kinship at all, but rather comes from *famulus,* "domestic slave."

This *familia,* then, is nearly the opposite of the "traditional" nuclear family – father, mother, and their kids, living as an economically independent unit. This is the model that social conservatives have often simply assumed in seeking to promote family values. So, too, have their liberal counterparts, who (apart from a few radical theorists) have usually taken the nuclear model as their starting point when seeking to expand its benefits to others such as "blended" households or same-sex couples.

Yet the Roman *familia* is closer to the Bible's understanding of family than the nuclear variety. In the Old Testament, the term that recent translations render as "family" is literally "house of the father": a multigenerational household including children and grandchildren as well as unrelated dependents. (Unlike Roman law, the Old Testament withholds from the *pater familias* life-and-death power over those in his charge.)

While a full discussion of the Bible's treatment of family is impossible here, two themes stand out. First, it's hard to overstate the centrality that scripture gives to the union of a man and a woman joined in "one flesh" for the bearing of children. This union plays a starring role right in the Bible's first pages; it forms the basis of the Decalogue's commandment to "honor father and mother"; and, in the prophetic books, it becomes a key symbol of God's relationship to Israel – a symbol extended in the New Testament to the relationship of Christ to his bride, the church.

Second, the Bible loves genealogies. Scripture's many recitations of begats attest that family doesn't just concern the living: it extends backward to long-dead ancestors, and

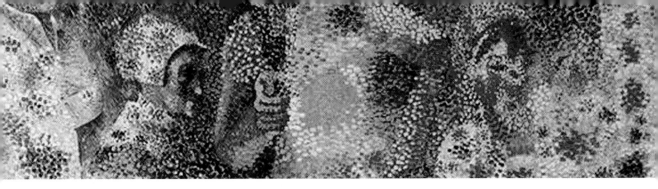

forward to unborn generations. "I don't know who my grandfather was; I am much more concerned to know what his grandson will be," Abraham Lincoln famously remarked, rejecting the notion that bloodlines matter. Scripture, by contrast, seems very much concerned to know who your grandfather was.

These twin scriptural themes may strike many as not just conservative, but downright archaic. Taken together, they insist that we do not make ourselves; instead, our families make us. We are not at liberty to choose our own identities and loyalties; our families give these to us.

Some Christians might wish to set these twin themes aside as historical side notes, like Leviticus's ban on eating shellfish. Inconveniently, however, both themes show up conspicuously in the New Testament. In two of the Gospel accounts, the greatest story ever told kicks off with genealogical tables seemingly cut-and-pasted from a first-century version of *Ancestry.com*. And lest anyone be tempted to dismiss the Adam and Eve story as an ancient myth reflecting outdated social norms, Jesus reaffirms it, emphatically and verbatim, in his startling words forbidding divorce. The lifelong union of one man and one woman, he teaches, is a unique bond sanctioned directly by God: "What God has joined together, let no man put asunder."

So far, so good for traditional family values. But Jesus, having reaffirmed the biological family, went on to deny it pride of place. Though he declared marriage divinely instituted, he remained celibate, praising those who "have made themselves eunuchs for the sake of the kingdom of heaven." As the scion of a royal lineage, he himself fathered no heir. Apparently contradicting the Decalogue, he commanded his disciples to "leave father and mother and come and follow me."

And he redefined the bonds of kinship: "Who is my mother, and who are my brothers? . . . Whoever does the will of my Father in heaven is my brother, and sister, and mother." The biological family, evidently, matters greatly; but in the order of our loves, it should come a distinct second. The care we owe our relatives remains, but now we're called to extend it to a vast new throng of siblings – a family of many ethnicities and cultures that includes the widowed, the unmarried, the outsider, and the stranger. As the early Christians showed, this mutual care must go beyond mere spiritual fraternity to include a degree of economic sharing that makes today's socialism seem weak beer. Family values of the Christian sort ought to make onlookers exclaim (in Tertullian's words): "See how they love one other."

This issue of *Plough* aims to reflect on what a family is, so that the transformations needed to solve the crisis of the family start from a firm basis, not a nostalgic ideal or progressive theorizing. And it seeks to explore what families are for. They aren't just good in themselves (though they undoubtedly are that too, not least as schools in the love of neighbor). More vitally, they are living symbols pointing to the truest of families: the kingdom of the Father of all. ⤜

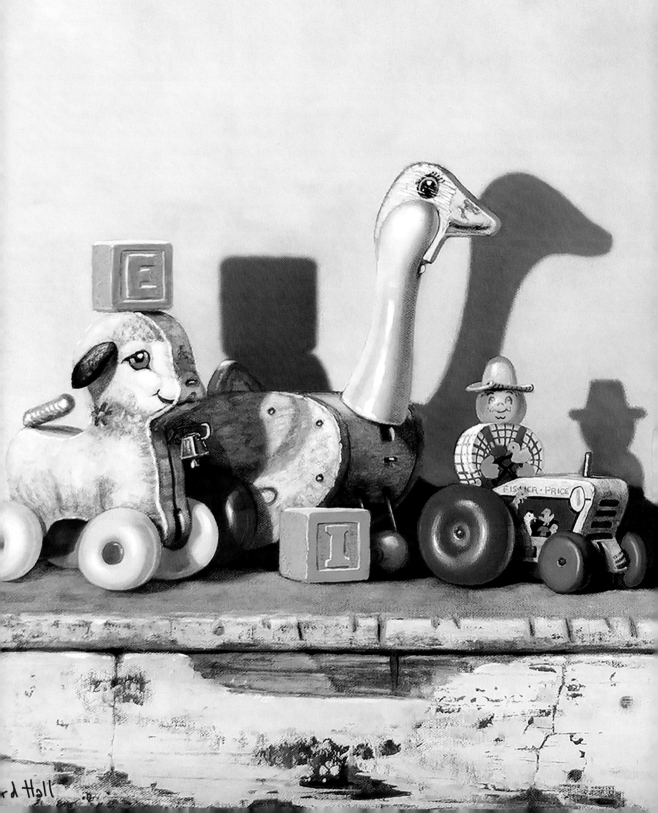

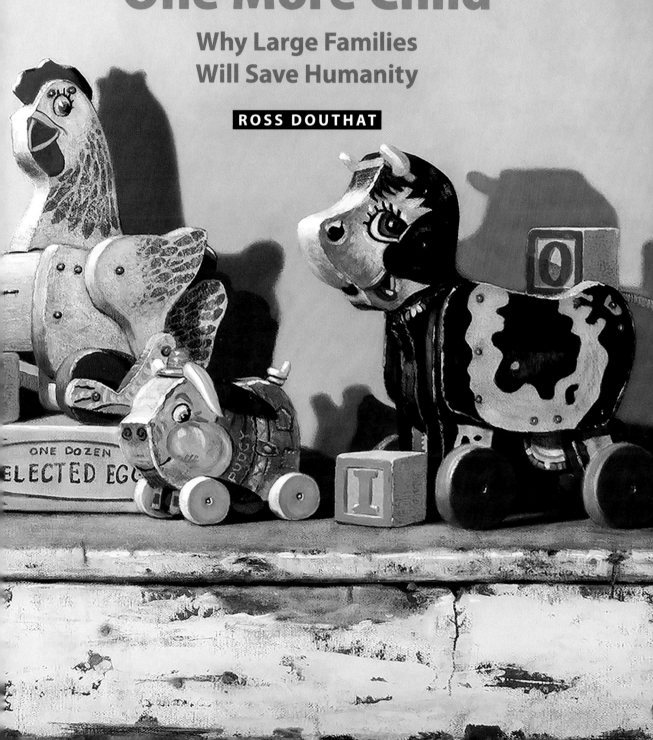

# The Case for One More Child

## Why Large Families Will Save Humanity

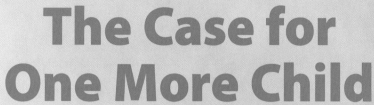

ROSS DOUTHAT

## Our society's future would be radically different if people simply had as many kids as they desired.

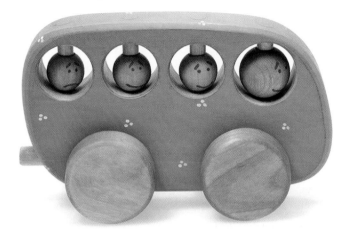

## What's stopping them?

**S**TART WITH THE CAR SEATS. They hulk in the back seats of any normal sedan, squeezing the middle seat from both directions, built like a captain's chair on *Star Trek* if James T. Kirk was really worried about taking neck damage from a Romulan barrage. The scenes of large-family life from early in the automobile era, with three or four kids jammed happily into the back seat of a jalopy, are now both unimaginable and illegal. Just about every edition of *Cheaper by the Dozen*, published

in 1948, uses an image of the Gilbreth kids packed into the family automobile, overflowing like flowers from a vase. Today, the car seats required to hold them would take up more space than the car itself.

In his 2013 book *What to Expect When No One's Expecting*, Jonathan V. Last described "car seat economics" – the expense and burden of car seats for ever-older kids, the penalties imposed on parents who flout the requirements – as an example of the countless "tiny

---

*Ross Douthat is a columnist for the* New York Times *and the author of several books, most recently* The Decadent Society: How We Became the Victims of Our Own Success *(Simon & Schuster, 2020).*

evolutions" that make large families rarer. Obviously car seats aren't as big a deal as the cost of college or childcare, or the cultural expectations around high-intensive parenting. But it's still a miniature case study, Last suggested, in how our society's rules and regulations conspire against an extra kid.

Seven years later, two economists set out to prove him right. In a paper entitled "Car Seats as Contraception," they argued that car-seat requirements delay and deter the arrival of third children, especially, because normal backseats won't hold three car seats, so you basically can't have a third young kid in America unless you upgrade to a minivan. The requirements save lives – fifty-seven child fatalities were prevented in 2017, the authors estimate. But they prevent far more children from coming into existence in the first place: there were eight thousand fewer births because of car-seat requirements in 2017, according to their calculations, and 145,000 fewer births since 1980.

You don't have to quite believe the specificity of these numbers to see that an important truth is being revealed. Our society is not exactly more hostile to children than societies in the past: indeed, once an American child is born, her girlhood will be safer from all manner of perils than the childhoods of the 1980s, let alone the farm-and-factory past. But this protectiveness coexists with a tacit hostility toward merely potential children – children who might exist, children who are imagined when people are asked about their ideal family size, but who, for all kinds of reasons, are never conceived or never born.

We lack a moral framework for talking about this problem. It would make an immense difference to the American future if more Americans were to simply have the 2.5 kids they say they want, rather than the 1.7 births we're averaging. But talking about a declining birthrate, its consequences for social programs or economic growth or social harmony, tends to seem antiseptic, a numbers game. It skims over the deeper questions: What moral claim does a potential child have on our society? What does it mean to fail someone who doesn't yet exist?

THINK ABOUT THIS with our daughter Rosemary, our fourth child, six months old as I write. We weren't sure if we could have her, or if we should. I had been sick with a debilitating illness that maybe – not officially, but definitely anecdotally – can be passed along to children. My wife carried the scars of several caesarean sections. We had moved three times in five years, losing money as we went. Much more than with any of her siblings, having Rosemary was a leap of faith.

She was conceived in the summer of 2019. In the winter of 2020, I brought Covid-19 home to my family from a book tour, and our other children and my seven-months-pregnant wife got sick. Rosemary was born amid the first wave of the pandemic; her birthday matches the exact late-April peak of deaths for our home state of Connecticut.

After we brought her back from the hospital, healthy and cheerful, I thought about what would have happened if news from 2020 had fallen back through a wormhole into 2019. *Guess what? Before you conceive another child, you should know that there will be a pandemic next year, the economy will shut down, there will be riots and a crime wave, and you'll all get sick with the virus, deep into your wife's pregnancy.* Would Rosemary have been conceived in the shadow of that foreknowledge? Would we have made the leap?

Because of course now that she is here she has inestimable value. How could the challenges of 2020, however dire they might

Previous spread: Richard Hall, *EIEIO*

have sounded as prophecy, possibly justify her non-existence? How could we not have pressed ahead, if the endpoint was her friendly cheeks, her babyish giggles, her oh-so-human eyes?

THE IDEA THAT not-enough-Rosemarys might be a problem for the world has taken a long time to take hold. The consensus during my youth held that falling birthrates were always a sign of progress, that Third World overpopulation might doom the world to famine, and that anyone who cared too much about Western fertility was probably a crank.

**The birthrate is entangled with any social or economic challenge that you care to name.**

I took this gospel for granted as a child: I remember quizzing my dad about how the earth could possibly survive the combination of overpopulation and pollution. But I also came young to the realization that the problem might lie elsewhere. Sometime in Bill Clinton's presidency, I was assigned a high school science bulletin-board project on population trends. In the library I checked out all the books on overpopulation – which meant basically the collected works of Paul Ehrlich, the alarmist author of *The Population Bomb*. When I compared their 1970s-era projections to what was actually happening, my teenage self could see two things plainly: first, none of the disasters Ehrlich envisioned had come to pass, and second, for the rich world the population trend was an arrow pointing down and down and down.

I was hardly the first person to notice this: P. D. James's dystopian prophecy of mass infertility, *The Children of Men*, came out five years before my bulletin-board revelation. But the fear of underpopulation belonged to the realm of weirdos and conservatives (but I repeat myself) well into my adulthood. When Hollywood got around to adapting James's novel in 2006, the film focused more on terrorist disturbances and cruelty to immigrants than the horror of a childless world. When countries in East Asia and then Eastern Europe began to search for policies to bolster birthrates, they were regarded as illiberal curiosities.

It was only when the US birthrate, long an above-average outlier among rich nations, began to descend anew following the Great Recession that the topic began to spark stirrings of real interest. But even now there's no agreement that the birthrate deserves as much attention as healthcare or taxes or abortion or police brutality, let alone that it might be one of the most pressing issues of our time.

Yes, Republicans can be induced to include a little family-friendly tax policy in a larger tax reform, and Democrats support family subsidies when they're cast as measures to fight poverty. But to argue that the American future depends on pushing our birthrate back above replacement level, as Matthew Yglesias did in his recent book *One Billion Americans*, remains an eccentric argument to many people: an interesting idea, maybe, but not a particularly urgent one, and certainly not the sort of issue that would make the cut of questions for a presidential debate.

WHICH IS A BIT CRAZY, when you stop to think about it. Whether a society is reproducing itself isn't an eccentric question; it's a fundamental one. The birthrate isn't just an indicator of some nebulous national greatness; it's entangled with any social or economic challenge that you care to name.

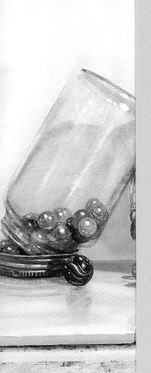
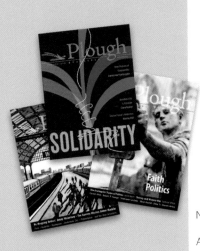
As social scientists have lately begun "discovering," a low-birthrate society will enjoy lower economic growth; it will become less entrepreneurial, more resistant to innovation, with sclerosis in public and private institutions. It will even become more unequal, as great fortunes are divided between ever smaller sets of heirs.

These are just the immediately measurable effects of a dwindling population. They don't include the other likely effects: the attenuation of social ties in a world with ever fewer siblings, uncles, cousins; the brittleness of a society where intergenerational bonds can be severed by a single feud or death; the unhappiness of young people in a society slouching toward gerontocracy; the growing isolation of the old.

Families can be over-sentimentalized, imprisoning, exhausting. But they supply goods that few alternative arrangements can hope to match. No public program could have replaced the network of relatives that helped my grandfather live independently until

his death – even if, yes, his five children, my mother and aunts and uncles, had often feuded with him and each other over the years. No classroom is likely to supply the education in living intimately with other human beings that my children gain from growing up together – even if the virtue of forbearance is not always perfectly manifest in their interactions.

*Yea, thou shalt see thy children's children, and peace upon Israel,* runs the Psalmist's blessing. A society of plunging birthrates withdraws the first blessing, and compromises the second day by day.

**B**UT TO IDENTIFY these problems is to run into a question: Whose responsibility, exactly, is it to fix them? One reason that the healthcare system and the tax code come up at presidential debates is that both involve official choices about how to regulate and spend. But the government cannot conjure babies (yet), and fertility decisions

Richard Hall, *Lost My Marbles*

belong to an intimate sphere that we rightly insulate from the reach of state coercion. And modern societies feel uncertain about whether they can even *ask* people to have kids, since that implies a moral obligation to have children.

Such an obligation was assumed by most peoples in human history, but most peoples were not us: freed from patriarchal demands, liberated from economic systems in which an extra pair of hands is an automatic asset, proud of the opportunities available to women, too secular to accept "be fruitful and multiply" admonitions, and conscious that there are eight billions of us and counting on an earth whose environment is, put mildly, under strain.

Still, even for a secular society it isn't hard to generate a moral-obligation-to-procreate case. You can just play the utilitarian game: Society should seek the greatest good for the greatest number; there is no good so essential as existence, so society should be organized to maximize, within reason, the number of people that exist.

I said *within reason* because that's how even the most child-friendly parents tend to

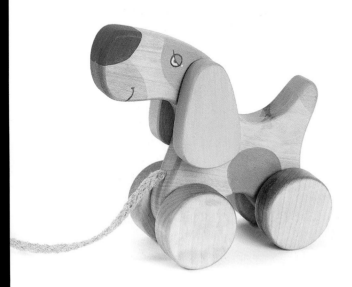

think. You have to go pretty deep into religious traditionalism to find people who don't do anything to space their children, and put their childbearing exclusively in the hands of God. The rest of us, even the people who embody what a *Washington Post* journalist once called "smug fecundity," tend to balance the number of kids they have against some other perceived good: not just health or the demands of some humanitarian vocation, but education, real estate, professional ambition. And, of course, the desire to someday get a little sleep.

But maybe this "reasonability" concession gives too much away. A famous rejoinder to the utilitarian case for more kids is that it leads to what the philosopher Derek Parfit termed the "Repugnant Conclusion" – namely, that so long as we consider existence itself a utilitarian trump card, we have to conclude that for "any possible population of at least ten billion people, all with a very high quality of life, there must be some much larger imaginable population whose existence, if other things are equal, would be better even though its members have lives that are barely worth living."

The supposed repugnance of this conclusion need not be conceded. The religious believer who regards suffering as freighted with potential moral purpose will have a very different reaction to a phrase like "barely worth living" than the typical secular utilitarian. The world of one hundred billion people who suffer tribulations might produce more saints; the world of ten billion people enjoying unparalleled hedonic pleasures might be under divine judgment.

Yet in framing the choice to have more kids as something that we should favor only *within reason*, aren't we tacitly embracing some version of Parfit's thesis – in the sense that for ourselves, we assume that there exists some family size whose possible tribulations exceed the good of an extra human being's existence? Aren't even we, the relatively fertile, minimizing our obligation to children yet unborn?

PERHAPS MEDIEVAL CATEGORIES can help us. Perhaps we can say that the unique sacrifices required of parents – and let's be clear that they're required of women more than men – make the absolute case for children a *counsel of perfection*, a marital equivalent to the chastity and poverty and obedience demanded of members of consecrated life. The family that is open to new life unstintingly, eschewing not just contraception but any kid-spacing caution, is living a supererogatory life, going beyond the basic requirements of the moral law, in a way that we should admire without feeling condemned if we cannot do the same.

Just how many kids would count as supererogatory under this moral theory is another question. Kid-spacing caution was invented long before the 1960s, but clearly people in the past wouldn't have regarded four or five kids as some sort of heroic, saintly, half-mad effort.

On the other hand, we shouldn't overestimate the gulf between past and present either. People in many premodern societies married later than historical clichés suggest, and infant mortality rates meant that how many kids you bore was tragically different from how many kids you raised. Raising five children to adulthood would have been very normal in, say, seventeenth-century New England, but raising a Quiverfull-style dozen would have been exceptional even then.

Since my wife and I obviously did some spacing of our children, I'm aware that the decision to have only a "reasonable" number can be driven by all kinds of non-saintly, self-justifying considerations. But the idea of reasonability definitely influences how I think about persuading *other* people, my more secular neighbors especially, that more kids would be better. I don't expect America to suddenly become filled with ten-kid families driving hulking vans. Rather, in a rich society with a plunging birthrate, the plausible goal should be to help more families have the kids they already say they want, meaning not six or eight or ten, but just one more – the kid who requires a new car seat and maybe a new SUV, the kid they feel like they might be able to afford, the kid you can feel pretty sure they won't regret.

**The goal should be to help more families have the kids they already say they want.**

SO WHAT KEEPS US from that one-extra-kid world? One answer is that too many people fear that the repugnant scenario is here already – that overpopulation and climate change will between them usher in a future of unparalleled misery.

"Meet Allie, One of the Growing Number of People Not Having Kids because of Climate Change," runs a recent NPR headline. Miley Cyrus recently declared her intention to refrain from procreating until somebody fixed the climate crisis: "I refuse to hand that down to my child."

I'm not sure I believe her, though. I know there are *some* people who are sincerely child-free because they fear the ecological impact of overpopulation. This strikes me as a deeply mistaken approach to the climate crisis – above all, because any long-term solution will require exactly the kind of human ingenuity that a stagnant gerontocracy will tend to smother. But I can concede that it has some coherence, some altruistic pull.

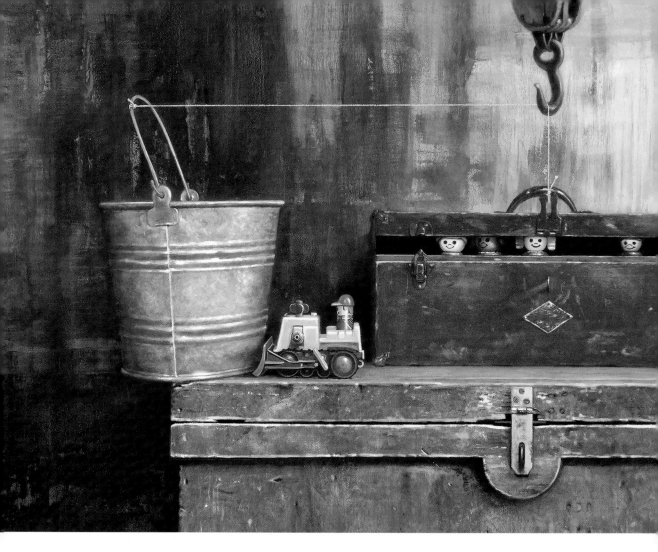

Richard Hall, *The Great Escape*

Those I doubt are the people claiming that they're refraining from having children for *the kid's sake*, in a reversal of the argument for a moral obligation to have kids. Humankind has existed this long because people have borne children under radically difficult circumstances, amid famine, war, and misery on a scale we can't imagine. Nothing in the potential life awaiting Miley Cyrus's hypothetical daughter promises hardship remotely comparable to those ancestral burdens. And even if you think climate change will be truly apocalyptic, it's no more threatening than the prospect of nuclear annihilation, which did nothing to prevent the last great Western baby boom.

No: In most cases, invoking climate anxieties seems more like an excuse, a gesture to ideological fashion, than a compelling explanation of low fertility. There has to be a deeper cause.

SO LET'S NAME THREE. First, romantic failure – not just in breakdowns like divorce, but in the alienation of the sexes from one another, the decline of the preliminary steps that lead to children, including not just marriage but sexual intercourse itself. Some combination of wider forces, the postindustrial economy and the sexual revolution and the identity-deforming aspects of the internet, are pushing the sexes ever more apart.

Second, prosperity, in two ways. One, because a rich society offers more everyday pleasures that are hard to cast aside in the way that parenthood requires. (Nothing gave me more sympathy for the childless voluptuaries of a decadent Europe than the first six months of caring for our firstborn.) Two, because prosperity creates new competitive hierarchies, new standards for the "good life," that status-conscious people respond to by delaying parenthood and having fewer kids.

Finally, secularization – because even if it's possible to come up with a utilitarian case for having kids, the older admonitions of Genesis appear to have the more powerful effect. The mass exceptions to low birthrates are almost always found among the devout, and the big fertility drop-offs in the United States correlate clearly with dips in religious identification.

The first of these three causes comes latest in history: the alienation of the sexes is mostly a post-1970s phenomenon, and previously any trend had run the other way. (More American women were married in the 1950s than in the 1880s.) Wealth and secularization, on the other hand, come in together centuries back, and entangle in all kinds of complicated ways.

In *How the West Really Lost God*, her provocative theory of secularization, Mary Eberstadt argues that the waning of the family led to declining religiosity rather than the other way around. Thus, for instance, the secularism of the Millennial generation might reflect their experience growing up as children of divorce, with weaker kinship networks leading to weaker ties to churches and other forms of communal life.

But I suspect it's wiser to see the whole process as a set of feedback loops: the rich society creates incentives to set aside faith's admonitions, which orients its culture more toward immediate material pleasures, which makes its inhabitants less likely to have children, which weakens the communal transmission belt for religious traditions, which pushes the society further along the materialist-individualist path. . . . and at a certain point you end up, well, here, with unparalleled prosperity joined to seemingly irresistible demographic decline.

S O HOW MIGHT IT be resisted? One answer is the kind of self-consciously reasonable vision I've already invoked – the push to just get back to replacement-level fertility, the push for one-extra-kid for families on the fence. The hope would be that the car-seat economists are right, and that simply by making family more afford-able – reducing the cost of childcare or of a parent staying home, reducing the cost of education, reducing the cost of home buying, and so on – you can change both the immediate incentives and the cultural expectations around having kids.

**Even if you think climate change will be apocalyptic, it's no more threatening than the prospect of nuclear annihilation, which did nothing to prevent the last great Western baby boom.**

The more it seems affordable to have a third or fourth child, in this hopeful theory, the more relaxed the whole culture might become – with less shaming of the fecund poor, less eyebrow-raising at large families in the upper middle class, and a lot more leniency for parents towing their broods on cross-country flights.

The more you deliberately organize institutions around supporting families, the more children would seem like a complement to education and opportunity rather than a threat.

And the more you take family formation seriously as a policy goal, the more you transcend certain fruitless culture wars, and move toward a world where more mothers work part-time or stay home while their kids are young *and* more fathers play the paternal role that made possible not just Ruth Bader Ginsburg's career, but Amy Coney Barrett's as well.

I have some hope in this vision, in part because I move back and forth between secular and Catholic worlds – from contexts where we're an oversize family to contexts where we're below-average wimps. And so far in the secular world I don't see all that much of the judging and hostility that some parents of large families report. (Though maybe the judging only kicks in once you have five or six.) Instead, I see a certain amount of friendly admiration, joined in people older than us to a mild *I wish we'd had three instead of two* regret.

> **For the average sinner, life with children establishes at least some of the preconditions for growing in holiness.**

Meanwhile, from the strange worlds of mommy bloggers and Instagram influencers all the way up to the Duggars of TLC, our pop culture manifests at least as much fascination with large families as it does with overpopulation fears. Maybe this fascination is itself a symptom of ill-health, a weird voyeurism about something that should come naturally. But at the very least it's an homage that sterility plays to fecundity, and a signifier that there are lots of people who might have more kids if their situation felt slightly different, if economic pressures changed and cultural expectations altered with them.

**A**GAIN, THAT'S WHAT I'd like to believe can happen. But there are still times, many of them featuring the overwhelming exhaustion you feel at the end of a professional-parental day, I think that no, to get *lots* more people to sign up for this kind of lifestyle, you would need something more than a "parenting more than two kids: it's more feasible than you think!" pitch. You would need our society to become dramatically unlike itself, ordered to sacrifice rather than consumption, and to eternity rather than what remains of the American Dream. You would need not change on the margins, but transformation – probably religious transformation – at the heart.

Certainly you can see the possible limits of policy tweaks and cultural nudges in the experience of other countries. The rich society that fully acknowledges an obligation to the unconceived may not exist, but many societies, European and Asian, do much more to support parents than the United States. And their results are not overwhelming: at the margins, policy can encourage births, but usually that means going from 1.4 kids per woman to 1.55, or 1.7 to 1.8 – gains that are fragile and easily swamped, both by specific events (like the Great Recession or the coronavirus) and by larger trends like the continued retreat from marriage and intimacy.

So perhaps a greater cultural change in what we *want* is needed, even for a goal as modest as a fertility rate that matches our professed desires. And this change might not actually start with (even if it would necessarily include) a renewed sense of obligation to generations yet unborn. Instead, it might start with what we the living want and seek out for ourselves.

The libertarian economist Bryan Caplan once wrote a book called *Selfish Reasons to Have More Kids*, which falls mostly into the nudging sales-pitch category: it's a list of reasons why

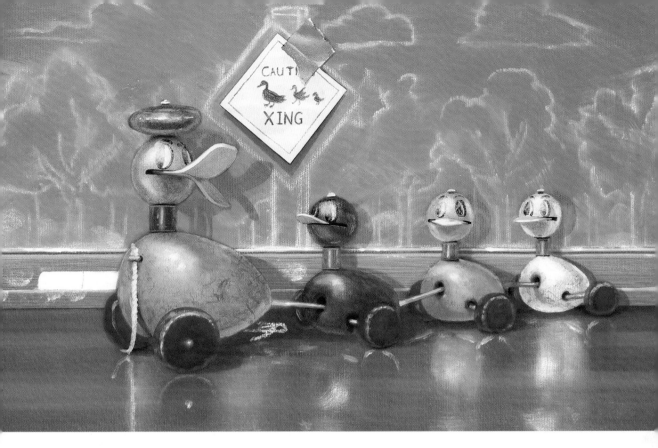

having a big family is more compatible with normal late-modern ideas of fulfillment than many people think.

The deepest reason to have more kids, though, is self-centered in a radically different way. It's that if you don't feel cut out for spiritual heroism, if you aren't chaste or poor or particularly obedient, if you aren't ready to be Mother Teresa – well, then having a bunch of kids is the form of life most likely to force you toward kenosis, self-emptying, the experience of what it means to live entirely for someone other than yourself.

This can circle back to egotism, admittedly, for people who make idols of their children or practice a ruthless selfishness toward everyone outside the charmed circle of their household. Jesus called us to leave behind fathers and brothers for a reason: it's still holier to be Francis of Assisi than a dad.

For the average sinner, though, for me and maybe for you, life with children establishes at least some of the preconditions for growing in holiness, even if there's always the risk of being redirected into tribal narcissism. If I didn't have kids there's a 5 percent chance that I'd be doing something more radical in pursuit of sainthood; there's a 95 percent chance that I'd just be a more persistent sinner, a more selfish person, because no squalling infant or tearful nine-year-old is there to force me to live for her and not myself.

But the idea of parenthood as enforced kenosis is very different from the idea that having more kids is swell and good and all-American. The large family as a spiritual discipline, children as a life hack that might crack the door of heaven – if that's the worldview required to make our society capable of reproducing itself again, then we're waiting not for child tax credits, better work-life balance, or more lenient car-seat laws, but for a radical conversion of our hardened modern hearts. ⤛

Richard Hall, *Duck Crossing*

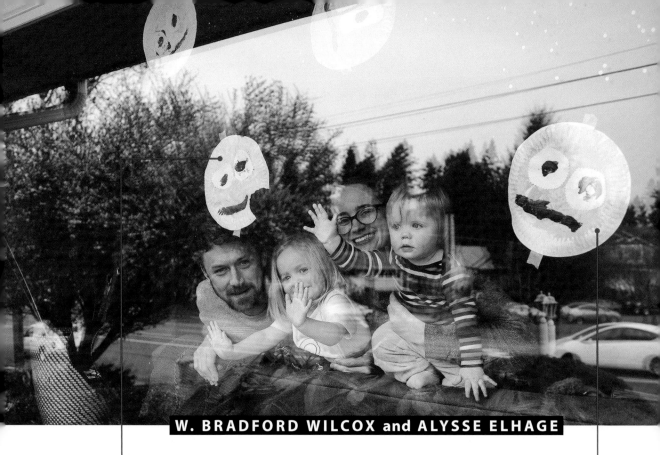

## W. BRADFORD WILCOX and ALYSSE ELHAGE

# The Best of Times, the Worst of Times

## *Family Life during Covid-19*

**T**HE COVID PANDEMIC and its effects – lost jobs, falling financial fortunes, deaths of family and friends, months stuck in isolation – have drastically changed the lives of billions. In the United States, poor and working-class people have been hit hardest, the Robert Wood Johnson Foundation reports. So how has all this turmoil affected the family?

When it comes to US family life in the time of Covid, media reports are mixed – perhaps the pandemic has made families stronger. Or weaker. Divorce is either falling or soaring. As for parents, especially those juggling jobs, child care, and online education, a recent American Enterprise Institute report concluded they are "not all right."

The American Family Survey (AFS) has released the first major report on family dynamics since the pandemic began, giving us an early look at the real state of family life during its first several months. The AFS report, from a nationally representative YouGov

---

*W. Bradford Wilcox is director of the National Marriage Project at the University of Virginia and a senior fellow of the Institute for Family Studies. Alysse ElHage is editor of the* Family Studies *blog.*

survey of three thousand Americans conducted in July 2020 by the *Deseret News* and the Center for the Study of Elections and Democracy, allows us to paint a complex picture that tracks closely with the increasingly unequal character of the nation.

First the good news:

## Stronger Families

Many marriages have emerged stronger from the pandemic, as couples turn toward one another for support. According to the AFS, 51 percent of husbands and wives (aged 18–55) say the pandemic has deepened their commitment to their spouse or partner, versus only 8 percent who disagree. A majority, 58 percent, also report that this year's challenges have made them appreciate their spouse more.

Families are also doing better in other ways. Unsurprisingly, married people in the survey were less likely to report loneliness than their single peers. More families report eating dinner together: up from 49 percent in 2019 to 54 percent in 2020. This is good news; eating dinner together several nights a week has been linked to better health and academic outcomes for children.

Finally, if we look at national trends, we see that the clear majority of children (about 60 percent) are being raised by their married biological parents. Even better, the share of children in intact families (with biological or adoptive married parents) has ticked upwards in recent years.

## Divorce Is Down and May Decline Further

More good news: couples who do get married are far less likely to divorce today than during the divorce revolution of the 1970s. In fact, divorce has been declining since the 1980s, dropping about 20 percent over the last decade to a point near the 1970 rate.

The AFS report indicates that the divorce rate is unlikely to rise because of Covid; the share of married people reporting trouble in their marriages has fallen from 40 percent in 2019 to 29 percent in 2020. (There was a similar pattern during the Great Recession, when divorce declined by 7 percent; some predict it will decline even further in the coming years.)

Americans also appear to have become less tolerant of divorce. Marriage is increasingly seen as a stable place to raise children, particularly for the college-educated, who are more likely to get and stay married.

## A Decline in Nonmarital Births

As a result of the pandemic and social distancing, unwed childbearing is likely to decrease. Like divorces, nonmarital births have been falling since the Great Recession, dropping from record highs: the rate of unmarried births decreased from 41 percent in 2009 to 39.6 percent in 2018. According to the AFS, singles reported having markedly less sex in 2020 than married individuals, with predictable consequences for 2021.

The good news about family in America, then, is that *a clear majority of marriages today will go the distance* and *the share of children being born and raised in stable marriages is rising.* All of this is great news for children and their families.

But there is some bad news that should trouble those concerned about the future:

## Stressed Families

Even as some families have grown stronger, the shutdowns, isolating conditions, and uncertainty of 2020 have placed enormous stressors on many, especially among those who suffered job or income loss. These economic blows have hit working-class and poor families hardest. Overall, about 34 percent of married Americans (18–55) in the AFS survey report that

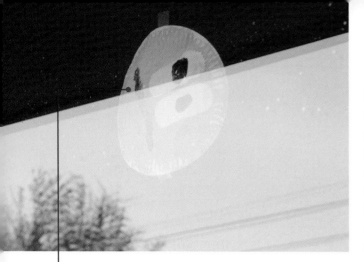

Covid has caused relationship stress. Not surprisingly, financial distress exacerbates problems: 45 percent of those who experienced falling finances say Covid has increased marital stress, versus 28 percent who experienced no financial crisis.

### Declining Marriage Rates

There are also indications that the marriage rate, already at a record low, will continue to decline as a result of the pandemic. According to the AFS, among unmarried Americans ages 55 and younger, 7 percent say they are postponing marriage due to Covid.

Moreover, sociologist Wendy Wang shows in a new Institute for Family Studies (IFS) research brief that the share of never-married Americans has reached a new high (35 percent) and is likely to increase further, as has been the case after previous recessions. And, as Lyman Stone recently reported at IFS, state-level marriage-license data show a decline this year (down 18 percent in Hawaii, 17 percent in Florida, 9 percent in Arizona, and 8 percent in Oregon, the four states with data available for the lockdown months).

This means a large minority of Americans will not enjoy the financial, practical, and emotional benefits of marriage and parenthood, at least for some time. This leaves them vulnerable to isolation and loneliness as they age, increasing their risk of illness and earlier death.

### More Inequality

Even worse, the bad news falls disproportionately upon the most vulnerable: the poor and the working class. America is increasingly divided by class when it comes to the structure and quality of family life, with marriage a luxury embraced by the highly educated and affluent, who are more likely to marry for life and raise their kids in marriage. Poor and working-class Americans are more likely to cohabit and raise their kids in less stable unions, with enormous consequences. As Nobel laureate Jim Heckman recently noted, "Household structure plays a major role in shaping US inequality. There is an inherent difference between single-parent households and two-parent households."

If we do nothing to address the growing marriage divide, which seems to have deepened in the wake of Covid, we will witness deepening economic and social inequality as the educated and affluent reap the myriad benefits associated with stable marriage – not just more money but greater happiness – while the less privileged are increasingly consigned to unhappy, unstable families or permanent singledom.

But it does not have to be this way. Policy changes – for example, ending the marriage penalty facing too many working-class families, and passing a child allowance that shores up shaky finances – would help. So would launching a national campaign supporting the "success sequence" that encourages young adults to address education, work, and marriage before having children. Nothing could be more important than bridging this divide. After all, your odds of growing up in a strong and stable family should not depend upon the size of your parents' bank account. ⇒

# Return to Vienna

## A Kindertransport Child Comes Home

**NORANN VOLL**

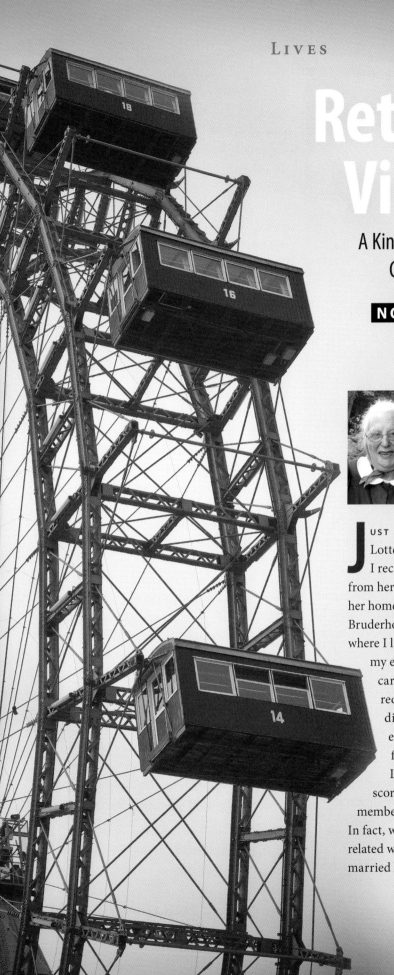

Lotte Berger Keiderling lost her mother in the Holocaust – and went on to bear thirteen children to "give Hitler a kick in the pants."

**J**UST DAYS BEFORE MY FRIEND Lotte Keiderling died in August, I received a handwritten card from her – the last of many sent from her home in an upstate New York Bruderhof to the Australian outback where I live. We'd been friends since my early twenties, when I helped care for her daughter Sonja, who required full-time care for her disability. We'd stayed in touch ever since – with her gift for friendship, at age eighty-nine Lotte still corresponded with scores of extended "family" members like me around the world. In fact, we'd recently become properly related when one of my nephews married her granddaughter; as I write,

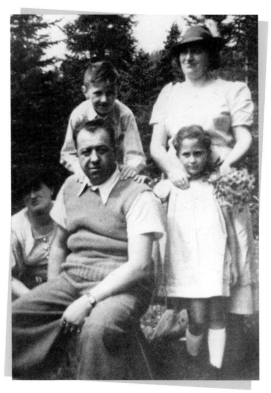

Lotte with her mother Valerie Berger *(right)* and her aunt, uncle, and cousin *(left)*, ca. 1934

child dreamed of riding – the tallest Ferris wheel in the world. She told of walking hand in hand with her father on Sunday afternoons along the Wiener Prater, into the Riesenrad-platz, where it stood. There, Lotte would beg her father to take her on the wheel.

"Please, Papi, please?"

But the answer was always the same: "Lottchen, when you are old enough I will take you. Not yet."

These precious memories comprised an entire childhood, condensed into a few short years. It ended abruptly, when she boarded a train without her parents; she didn't return for eight decades.

BY AGE SEVEN, after the 1938 *Anschluss*, Lotte had watched Hitler screech from a swastika-emblazoned balcony to adoring throngs shouting "Heil Hitler!" Not long after, she was chased down the streets by boys shouting "Jew! Jew!" Her parents had their bakery confiscated; she remembered her father refusing the nightly demands from bands of roving Nazis that he clean the pub across the street.

In June 1939, sensing impending doom, Josef and Valerie Berger put their much-loved seven-year-old daughter onto the lifesaving *Kindertransport* train with a small suitcase, a blanket, and her favorite foods. Where she was going, they told her, there would be horses (Lotte imagined the Lipizzaners of Vienna's Spanish Riding School). They promised that they would soon follow.

Lotte rode the train with hundreds of other weeping children, and, after a brief reconnection with relatives in London, was welcomed into the Cotswold Bruderhof, which had

I'm holding their baby, Ava, Lotte's great-granddaughter, in my non-writing arm.

But I only understood why Lotte so deeply treasured her family, both biological and adopted, when in 2018 she made a trip back to Vienna. She had always described her childhood hometown in vivid terms: a wonderland of promenades lined with horse-chestnut trees where she and her father gathered conkers; world-class musicians and Strauss waltzes; delicious *Torten*. She told of holidays in the Alps, ice cream by the Danube, and enough love from two adoring parents to overflow the heart of any child. As an adult, she could still sing the folksong her father had taught her: *"Nun ade, du mein lieb' Heimatland"*: "Farewell, my beloved homeland."

Above all, she remembered the mysterious Ferris wheel, or *Riesenrad*, every Viennese

*A farmer's daughter from New York, Norann Voll lives at the Danthonia Bruderhof in rural Australia with her husband, Chris, and three sons. She blogs at Bruderhof.com on discipleship, motherhood, and feeding people.*

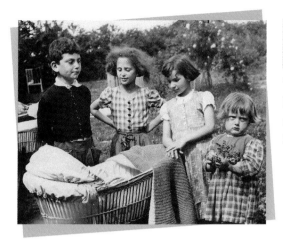

offered to take in four children fleeing Nazi persecution.

On arriving, Lotte stared: "All these women in kerchiefs and long dresses. I thought I'd landed on a different planet." And yet she soon felt at home, in what she described as "an atmosphere of love."

Even so, Lotte cried herself to sleep many nights as she thought of her parents. The threat of Nazism was never far away; later she remembered playing in the English meadows and seeing the familiar black cross on low-flying German planes overhead.

In 1941, when Bruderhof communities in England were ordered to emigrate to South America or face internment, the other three *Kindertransport* children at the community were returned to relatives. But after Josef and Valerie were asked whether Lotte should leave England for Paraguay, they wrote back immediately: "Take her as far away from Hitler as possible."

In the Paraguayan jungle, as the community struggled to build up a pioneering settlement, Lotte enjoyed what she described as a happy childhood, as a foster child with several families. Still, she craved the touch of her own mother. Once, a friend's mother noticed she was sad and took her onto her lap to comfort her, a moment Lotte cherished the rest of her life.

D URING THE FIRST YEAR IN Paraguay, Lotte received frequent letters from her parents, who were still in Vienna. Then the letters stopped. Time passed, and her parents became an increasingly distant memory. But in July 1945, a letter arrived from her father, postmarked Bergen-Belsen:

> My dearly beloved child,
> You will surely have joy in receiving a letter from your Papa. I hope you are well, which is the case with me. I have not heard about the whereabouts of your dear Mutti, as everyone had to travel with this war. I hope to see you soon; I want to either come to you or Uncle Adolf. Please write back immediately.
> Many thousand kisses from your Papa.
> Many greetings to Lene [Schulz, Lotte's guardian] and your schoolmates and Mr. Trümpi [her teacher].

Shortly after this brief note arrived, Lotte's teacher took her on a walk and told her that her mother was dead. The news had come from the doctor who had treated her father on his release from Bergen-Belsen – he had weighed only one hundred pounds, the doctor said. Lotte wept bitterly.

She and her father began to correspond. In May 1948, he wrote from a small town in Bavaria:

> My dearest Lotte!
> I received your dear letter from April 16, and was so happy about it. I am reassured if you write to me regularly. I wish I could mail you the wristwatch which I promised to you.
> As you do not remember Harry Raab I am sending you a photo of him today, which you and your dear Mutti are also on. At that time we were visiting you in the children's home in Annaberg. Please save this picture; it is precious. I got it from Aunt Carla.
> Do you still remember when I taught you to ride a small bike? It is nice to do some

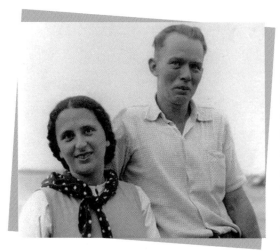

Roland and Lotte returning from their honeymoon; Paraguay, 1952

sport. I also ride my bike sometimes. Do you remember when we went ice skating? Perhaps the time will come when we can do this together again. It is very hot here now; always when I see the children eating ice cream I think of you, as I know how much you liked it too.

Now, my dear child, you will soon have your seventeenth birthday, and I want to wish you the very best for this day. May all your wishes be fulfilled and may you always stay healthy and happy. May God also grant me the joy that after so many years of separation I could embrace you once more.

On this day please think of your Papa who is so far away from you.

Josef's wish was never fulfilled. He eventually immigrated to the United States, where he settled in Niagara Falls, New York. Both dreamed of a reunion, but travel between Paraguay and the United States was a formidable economic obstacle, and before they could meet again, he died.

In the meantime, Lotte had reached adulthood, and in 1950, at age nineteen, she fell in love. It was a story she never tired of telling: "Roland was a German, but he didn't worry or care that I was Jewish. He just loved me, and I loved him. We married in 1952, and – guess what! – we had thirteen kids. So I say, 'I gave Hitler a kick in the pants!'"

Lotte's love for Roland and his for her began to heal the wound of loss that had accompanied her through childhood. Years later, she would write about the first afternoon after their honeymoon, when they settled into their first tiny one-room apartment. "We sat at our table and I just wept, because now we had our own home. Since leaving my parents as a young child, I had not had a home that was really my own – I was always cared for by other families. Having our own little home meant a great deal to me, and I kept it like a little jewel box, always with fresh flowers and just beautiful."

One baby followed the next. Sonja, their third, was born in 1957, healthy, brown-eyed, and robust at ten pounds. They were still living in Paraguay. When she was five months old, what began as an ear infection turned into severe meningitis. Despite being flown to Asunción for treatment, Sonja almost died, suffering severe brain damage. She was never able to talk, walk, or care for herself. Lotte, and later her other children with her, devoted herself to Sonja for the next forty-one years, until her death in 1998.

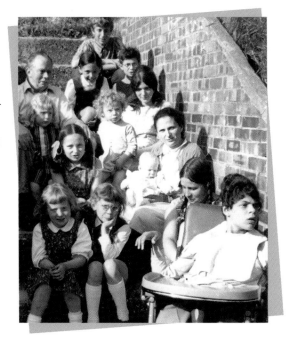

Shortly before immigrating to the United States: Lotte and Roland with twelve of their children in 1971, including Sonja (front)

By this time, Lotte's other eleven daughters and her son were grown, and many were having families of their own. Today her eighteen grandchildren and six great-grand-children live in the United States, Europe, and (in the case of baby Ava's family) here in Australia.

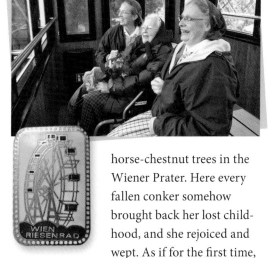

I N 1994, ROLAND AND LOTTE, long settled in New York, visited the Holocaust Memorial Museum in Washington, DC, to register her mother's name, hoping this might help bring to light more information about her imprisonment and death. Not long afterward, a hand-delivered letter from the American Red Cross finally gave a few sketchy details. Valerie Berger had been deported from Vienna to the Litzmannstadt (Łódź) Ghetto, in Poland, on October 19, 1941; barely six months later, on May 7, 1942, she died. Lotte was immensely grateful to learn the date her mother died, but the bare facts left a great deal to the imagination, and Lotte often found herself hoping that her passing had been natural and dignified.

In 2018, Lotte decided she would return for a visit to Vienna. Now eighty-seven and a widow (Roland had died in 2000), she wanted to see the city of her childhood. Finally, the folksong of farewell that her father had taught her was reversed.

As she and the daughters who traveled with her walked the streets of her beloved hometown, drank cream-topped coffee, and stood outside her parents' bakery and the family home, she connected to her *Heimatland* and its people. Strangers who heard her story prepaid her taxi fare. Others refused to let her pay for a meal, or for studio photos or souvenirs. A principal at a local high school invited her to speak to his students.

A particular moment of restoration came as she strolled down her favorite avenue of horse-chestnut trees in the Wiener Prater. Here every fallen conker somehow brought back her lost childhood, and she rejoiced and wept. As if for the first time, she could fully reflect on her parents' pain and suffering, and her own.

And, of course, she rode the *Riesenrad*; her eighty-year-old question, "Papi, when?" finally had its answer. One of her daughters told me later that it was a moment of pure, carefree wonder. As Lotte was carried high above the city that loved and betrayed her, the great wheel became a symbol of closure; a life came full circle in a union of completion and peace. Perhaps her father was there in the gondola with her.

Finally riding the *Riesenrad*: Lotte and her daughters Christine and Moni, 2018

B UT THE VISIT TO VIENNA was a continuation of Lotte's story, not its end. Among the Austrians she met were two women, Uta Lang and Marie-Louise Weißenböck, committed to working for reconciliation regarding the atrocities committed against Austria's Jews. After Lotte returned home, they arranged for researchers to investigate who Josef and Valerie Berger had been, and what had happened to them.

A year after the trip, Lotte learned that her parents had been deported together to Poland. This was welcome news – she had always

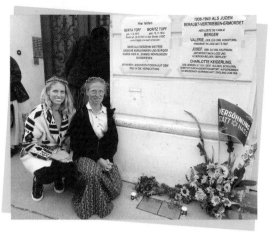

Dedication of the *Stolperstein:* Christine and Lotte's granddaughter Susanna, September 2020.

supposed they were separated right from the beginning, because of her father's letter from Bergen-Belsen, so she took some comfort in knowing they had spent her mother's last six months together.

More details followed. It emerged that the Bergers had not been bakers, as Lotte had always assumed; her mother had owned a bakery, while her father had worked in finance. Other researchers tracked down the Bergers' address in the Litzmannstadt ghetto, which allowed them to surmise how Valerie had died. She was, they determined, among the thousands of physically unfit inhabitants of the ghetto rounded up in early May 1942 to "ease overpopulation." They had all been gassed in mobile extermination vans.

When Lotte's daughter Christine called her with the news, she wept: "They killed my beloved mother!" Yet even in this fresh grief, she told her family, she was thankful to finally know the truth. She reflected:

> I learned how hate and selfishness can rule over a person such as Hitler and totally ruin the lives of millions of people. I also learned how important it is to uncover the fascinating stories that people can tell about amazing happenings, which are the foundations of history itself.

Back in Vienna, Uta Lang was working to make sure the memory of Lotte's family would be preserved. In recent decades, tens of thousands of distinctive *Stolpersteine* – brass "stumbling stones" with engraved names – have been installed in sidewalks or roadways outside the last freely chosen home or workplace of Jews and other victims of the Holocaust. The idea is metaphorical: they serve as figurative stumbling blocks for passersby, inviting reflection and keeping memories alive. A stone for Lotte's family was commissioned, to be installed outside her childhood home. The dedication date, initially set for May 2020, was postponed to September 27, 2020, because of the Covid-19 pandemic.

Lotte looked forward to the *Stolperstein* dedication with great anticipation, and wrote out a statement:

> I want to express my deep thankfulness to my dear parents Josef Berger, my father, and Valerie Berger, my mother, who in very dangerous times of Nazi persecutions not only against them personally, but against all Jewish people, including children, had the courage to send me, their only daughter, alone to safety in England, in June 1939.

One month before the ceremony, however, Lotte died. The family painted the Riesenrad on the lid of her pinewood coffin.

Christine attended the *Stolperstein* dedication in her mother's stead, together with a few dozen other relatives and friends. At Lotte's request, those present sang together the words of the prophets Isaiah and Micah, set to an ancient Jewish melody:

> Into plowshares turn their swords,
> nations shall learn war no more.
> And every man 'neath his vine and fig tree
> shall live in peace and unafraid.

"I felt Mama there with us," Christine told me. "She now knows perfect peace, and she was with us as we sang." ⤳

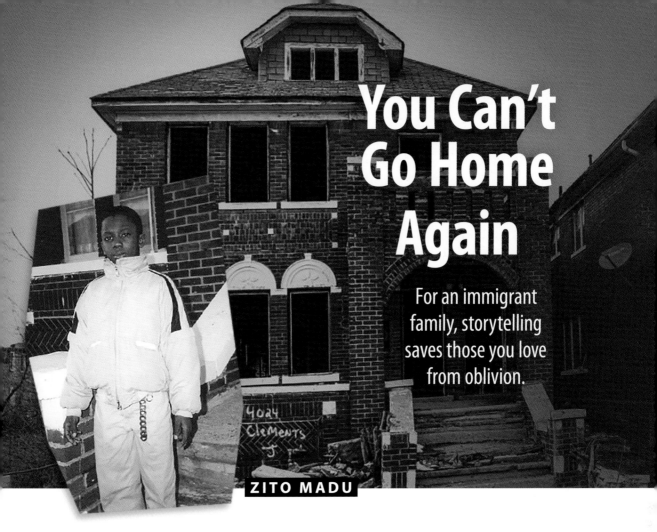

# You Can't Go Home Again

For an immigrant family, storytelling saves those you love from oblivion.

**ZITO MADU**

The author in front of his family's first house in Detroit (collage)

**M**Y FATHER LOVES TO TELL the story of the time my older brother and I got lost coming home from a festival in a neighboring village. We grew up in a remote Nigerian village in Imo State, and though the gathering was within walking distance, it's very dark at night out in the countryside.

My brother and I stayed at the festival much longer than we should have. By the time we began walking home, it had become difficult to see, and it was pouring rain. Maybe out of fear, or frustration, or simply because I was a difficult child, I eventually quit walking and sat down in the rain to cry.

My father, sensing that something was wrong, got on his motorcycle and set out to search for us. He rode around both villages, asking people if they had seen us. Eventually he found us on the side of the road. We rode back in the rain, my brother in the back and me clinging to my father's neck.

When my father tells the story, he does it in such detail that it seems as if he has just lived that day. He remembers the festival we went to, how long we were gone, what time it was when he started being worried, the people he spoke to, the road he found us on. It's as if he took detailed notes, yet there's no notebook or recording of the event. He can simply recall it whenever he wants.

It's not just his personal history and experiences that he recalls in such detail: our culture is passed along orally, and my father is a great storyteller. He has an almost encyclopedic

---

*Zito Madu is a writer living in Detroit, a contributor to* GQ, *and an avid lover of poetry.*

knowledge of our village and our people. He knows the branches of families, their beginnings and entanglements. He knows the true histories of many of the villagers and the myths that have determined the village's collective identity. Much of the information was passed down to him, but the rest he acquired on his own, listening and watching.

I envy his memory, as I can barely remember anything. I have a theory that the difference between us is that he is a person of community, and I am not. He thrives when surrounded by people and is uncomfortable in isolation. I choose to spend most of my time alone; it suits my nature. Solitude seems as if it should be suited to better memory, but it's had the exact opposite effect. With no one to remember with, my memories tend to wither, leaving only broad outlines, and my brain constructs false memories to fill in the gaps.

> **I envy my father's memory, as I can barely remember anything. I have a theory that the difference between us is that he is a person of community, and I am not.**

I often ask my father to document the things that he remembers about our village and our family. He tends to agree, but never follows through. He has no need to write his memories down, because he has no fear of forgetting them. The request is secretly for me, both because I want to learn more about who we are, and because I know that I'm already forgetting so much.

RECENTLY I BOUGHT SOME FILM to take pictures of the first house my family lived in when we moved to the United States in 1998; all eight of us lived in a single room on the second floor.

Encountering our landlord, Mr. Collins, was a saving grace. We had moved to Detroit

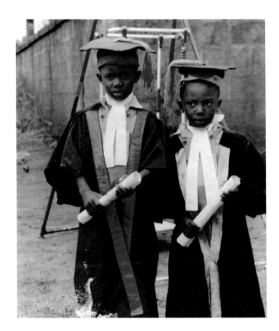

for the Nigerian community, but as my mother tends to put it, "we were utterly abandoned" after we arrived. Mr. Collins allowed us to live in that room rent-free for the first few months, and when he found out that we all used to huddle around the sole space heater at night, he brought us cold-weather clothes that had belonged to his family.

Mr. Collins had a wife named Cookie and a son and daughter. The son lived on the first floor of the same house we were in for some time, but he struggled with drug addiction. Once, he fought my father after my father refused to give him money under Mr. Collins's orders. Eventually the son moved out, first to another house nearby, and then he disappeared from the street and regular conversation. The daughter was better off. We saw her infrequently, but she was usually doing well.

Mr. Collins and his family provided us with small joys and relief in those harsh early years. They couldn't erase the pressures of poverty and acclimating to a new world, but he and his wife tried to alleviate them as much as they could. Sometimes it was allowing us to skip rent, other times it was taking the children for ice cream or to ride horses.

Mr. Collins and Cookie took me and my siblings to our first circus. They bought us toy lightsabers. When my father went from Rite Aid stock boy to a different schedule as a wineseller, Mr. Collins began to pick us up from school. He would take us to Belle Isle, the island park in Detroit. I still have a picture from that time of me standing on the top of its iconic big slide. I know without seeing him in the photo that Mr. Collins was waiting at the bottom. He and Cookie helped us have a childhood when we could have been crushed by the struggles of the new world.

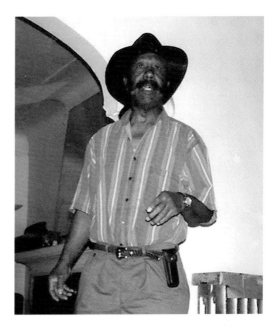

Mr. Collins in his younger days on a visit to the author's family

**A**FTER WE MOVED OUT and into our own house, we barely saw Mr. Collins anymore. Even though he was just a few miles away, the days seemed to press relentlessly against each other and there was so much chaos with everyone growing up and dealing with school and young adulthood. He came over periodically at first, but soon his own problems got too big as well. Somehow, though, my father seemed to stay in touch.

I was with my father when I last saw Mr. Collins and Cookie, who had dementia. The disease set on her and took over quickly. She didn't recognize us, and she barely recognized her husband. Watching his wife wither, taking care of her as she grew even more distant from him, had a visceral effect on Mr. Collins. Stress stripped his body down to a skeleton, and he swam in the same clothes that had been tight on him before.

Cookie died soon after our visit. About a year later, my father asked me if I wanted to go see Mr. Collins with him. I declined. I never got to see him again; soon Mr. Collins died as well.

I refused that final chance to visit because I wanted to avoid seeing him reduced by his troubles. I ran away from that encounter, but when I went to take pictures of the old house, connected so much to him and Cookie and the life they gave to it and us, I realized I was trying to capture what that first American home meant to me, to use photography as a tool of preservation. The house existed in a particular way in my imagination and I wanted to import it into memory, to translate it into something lasting. But all I saw was sadness and vanishing.

Time had done to the house what time does to everything. The essence of it had been washed away. I didn't want to take pictures of it, or even to stand and look at it. After all the house had meant, it felt unjust to document its ruin. The same went for the man who owned the house.

Sometimes I feel as if I write as a form of excavation, an act of finding. But it's inadequate for preserving the existence of the people and places I love – no number of words, however beautifully arranged, could ever revive their fullness. The irony is that the more I try, the more hollow and inadequate the result. In the face of this injustice, it almost seems that to be forgotten is better.

At the end of Julio Cortázar's 1949 play *The Kings*, the dying Minotaur insists that he does not want to be remembered. "A lifetime of forgetting awaits you," he tells his uncomprehending audience. "I don't want tears; I don't want statues. I only want oblivion. Only then will I be more myself." I imagine this recrimination coming from the people and places I try and fail to recover.

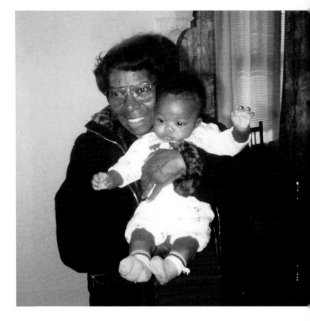

ABOUT THE TIME MR. COLLINS died, my father told me that one of my cousins in Nigeria had died as well. "Cousin" might not be the technically correct term for how Chuks and his family are connected to me; village families are linked in so many ways that it's difficult to untangle the details. Such an exercise is also unnecessary. He was my family.

Chuks was the youngest of six. His family had lived in a house in front of ours for generations and within that greater family, we also had generational friendships. Our own particular group of friends was my older brother and me, Chuks, and his two older brothers.

All we used to do in those days was play around. I barely remember school, but I remember playing soccer, playing by the school and church across the road from our homes, running through the fields at night to catch crickets, chasing bats from old buildings, and going to festivals together. My mother likes to remind me that whenever we all played, Chuks came home last – he lagged behind carrying the clothes and shoes that the rest of us had abandoned.

Years after we left, Chuks joined the church. He wanted to become a priest. He was walking home from Mass one night when he was killed; thieves hit him over the head with a blunt object. His body was found on the side of the road the next morning.

Chuks's death gave me a double shock. The first was at the sudden finality of death. No matter how common that great catastrophe is, it still remains absurd to me. That someone can be present in the world and then not, especially through a ridiculous chance – that he was in the wrong place at the wrong time – seems so cruel and unacceptable. Now, with so many vanishing due to the pandemic, the grief is repeated and unfathomable; that so many people in the world can disappear so quickly and irretrievably is overwhelming.

The second shock came when I realized that I couldn't remember his face. I had always taken joy in the fact that even though I hadn't seen him in a while, he existed somewhere, struggling and striving, being and becoming, that he and his goodness were present in the world. When he died, not only did I feel the grief of losing that joy, it became apparent that my memory of him was vanishing. I couldn't fully construct him anymore.

Almost ten years after leaving my old village, I went back to visit for the first time. When I arrived, it became evident that it wasn't just Chuks I was forgetting. There was a natural sense of familiarity, but so much of

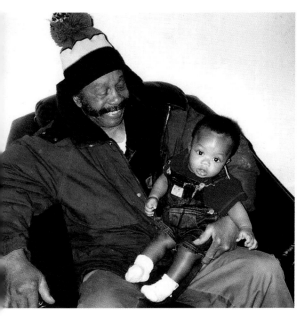

Mr. Collins with the author's younger sibling

W. S. Merwin once said about memory, noting this etymology. "Homecoming is what we all believe in. I mean, if we didn't believe in homecoming, we wouldn't be able to bear the day." Forgetting means that I can't go home, and that even at home in the village, I still feel far away.

That I can't hold on to the people and places I cherish feels as if I am losing who I am. Worse, if I can't remember them, I cannot testify to my love for them. In *Adam Bede*, George Eliot wrote: "Our dead are never dead to us until we have forgotten them: they can be injured by us, they can be wounded; they know all our penitence, all our aching sense that their place is empty, all the kisses we bestow on the smallest relic of their presence."

My father has no need to write down his memories and probably never will. I think that as a community man, he understands that he is part of a larger story and a collective memory that is contained with him but also supersedes him. He has no fear that the story will disappear with him, because the story is the people as a whole.

In my own alienation from that collective memory, I find myself excavating graves to bring things back to the surface. The anecdotes I can muster don't do them any more justice than the shards and bones of an archaeological dig do the fullness of the past. But in the process, I can at least bestow kisses on the smallest relic of their presence.

I never imagined becoming a writer, but now I write ghost stories out of desperation and hope against time and memory. It's an impossible hope, but it's one that I need in order to go home again. ➤

> **That I can't hold on to the people and places I cherish feels as if I am losing who I am.**

the place where I grew up felt alien, as if things were slightly askew. I saw people I should have known but couldn't remember, and I walked down roads I was sure I had been on before but couldn't place. It felt as if my full memories of the place and its people were just slightly out of view, that all I needed to do was to focus hard enough and turn toward them. But as much as I tried, the full picture never returned. Naturally, my father had none of those problems and fit back in as if he had never left.

I spent most of my time sitting and talking with Chuks's older sister, Chigozie, the last of his siblings who was still there. I told her stories of America, and she filled me in on what had happened since we left. Every morning I walked over to their house and sat with her until the evening, listening to her tell stories as I attempted to restore my memory of the place. The next time I went home, she had also left. I spent most of that visit confined to our house.

THE WORD *NOSTALGIA* COMBINES the Greek roots for "return home" and "pain" – a painful homecoming. "What we think of as the present is made up of the past," the poet

# Two Poems by Rachel Hadas

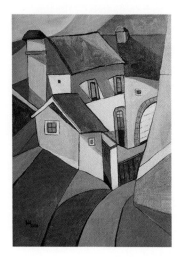

Aniko Hencz,
*Steep Street,*
acrylic on
canvas

## Trying to Get to School

Dream: halfway to my destination
I remembered something I'd forgotten
and turned around so I could get
it back before it was too late.

But making my way from A to B
could not be managed easily.
Locked courtyard, blocked alleys, a high wall –
I had to cross or climb them all.

I tried and tried without success.
Wherever I turned: NO ACCESS,
no way to reach the subway station
and get from there to my destination

across the river and into a room
I'd open the door to (what was Zoom?),
Enter, talk, listen, and engage
with my students, forgetting age,

and tell them, before time ran out,
what reading and writing were about.
Gathered together in one place,
to talk and listen, face to face:

this, my dream was telling me,
was something that could no longer be.
Henceforth it wouldn't be allowed
to be part of any crowd.

Locked courtyards and blocked alleyways,
our isolated nights and days,
no hands held up or questions asked,
the eager faces muffled, masked,

all siloed in our separate spaces,
and interposed between us: stasis.
I knew already there was no
way to get where I had to go.

The dream I dreamed six months ago:
Prophetic, but no longer true.
Now crowds have gathered – still masked, yes,
but shouting against voicelessness.

The streets are full, the atmosphere
ardent, infectious. Where is fear?
Forgotten in the hope and flow.
Justice is a pandemic too.

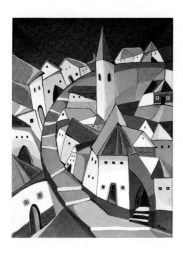

Aniko Hencz,
*The Street with
Many Stairs,*
acrylic on
canvas

## Lyric Leap

The fizzing spark, the lateral leap,
the sideways skitter (mind the gap!),
fugitive dream recalled mid-morning,
déjà vu pouncing without warning,
unexpected recollection,
serendipitous digression
meandering at an angle – pun
that stops you before you've begun,
tattered palimpsest, hapax,
puzzle that stymies you in your tracks,
lacuna, hiatus, sidebar,
sudden swerve, and you are far
along already toward surprise.
Pause a second and surmise.
Your destination was – where?
One sideways step may get you there,
your wings still crumpled, half asleep –
one unassuming lyric leap. ❧

The Unchosen
Obligations of
Family

# Why
# Inheritance
# Matters

An Interview with
Cardinal Christoph Schönborn

# Cardinal Schönborn, archbishop of Vienna, talks with *Plough*'s Kim Comer about family history, celibacy, monument toppling, and the healing of memory.

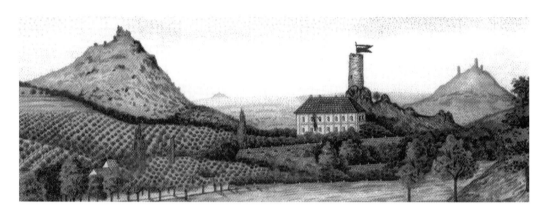

Skalka Castle, birthplace and ancestral castle of Cardinal Schönborn

*Previous spread:* Portraits of Cardinal Schönborn's ancestors

**Plough:** The child Christoph Maria Michael Hugo Damian Peter Adalbert Graf von Schönborn was born at Skalka Castle in 1945 and entered the world laden with a certain status and certain expectations. Did this inheritance ever seem oppressive?

**Cardinal Schönborn:** I was just nine months old when we were forced to leave our family castle in Bohemia, along with the other two million ethnic Germans expelled from Czechoslovakia after World War II. The next time I was inside a castle owned by my family, I was eighteen. In the meantime, I lived very far from castles, as the child of a refugee family – mostly we stayed with relatives who put us up here and there.

It's true that I was born into a family where certain things were expected of me, but I was the second son. My older brother would have inherited the family's estates according to the rules of *fideicommissum* succession, under which the oldest son is the sole heir to avoid splintering the inheritance. My mother used to tell how, when I was born, the midwife held me up and said, "Poor little thing, you get nothing but the garden!" As it turned out, because of our family's expulsion, I didn't even get the garden.

Still, from early on, I was interested in my family history. I discovered that the great careers of members of the Schönborn family were always in the Church. I had no way of knowing that I would become the eighth bishop and the third cardinal in our family's history.

These ancestors did not always act in accordance with our contemporary values. This past summer, around the world we saw monuments toppled because of the sins of the supposed heroes of the past. How do you view this?

I'll answer by giving examples from my own family. The first bishop in the family was Johann Philipp Schönborn, who in the 1600s served as

---

*Christoph Schönborn*, OP, is a friar, theologian, and the Cardinal Archbishop of Vienna. *Kim Comer* is editor of Plough's German-language edition.

archbishop of Mainz and bishop of Würzburg, and later of Worms as well. Though baptized a Protestant, he oversaw three bishoprics. By virtue of being archbishop of Mainz, he was also an imperial elector and the imperial archchancellor, charged with overseeing the election of a new Holy Roman Emperor. What did it mean to be both a bishop and a territorial prince, a spiritual and a secular leader at the same time?

This Johann Philipp lived through the misery of the Thirty Years' War, which decimated the population of Central Europe. On becoming archbishop and imperial chancellor in 1647, his most pressing concern was peace. He made decisive contributions to the Peace of Westphalia, which ended the war the following year. For this, he compromised with the Protestants – so much so that the papal nuncio in Germany, who later became Pope Alexander VII, criticized him for being overly conciliatory. But Johann Philipp, looking back on three decades of war, understood the great good of peace – and that for peace to last, the precondition was mutual tolerance.

Of course, today it's easy to see the defects in the Peace of Westphalia, which enshrined the principle of *cuius regio, eius religio* – the ruler of a territory determines its religion. This principle not only created peace, but also resulted in mass expulsions: Protestants were driven from Catholic areas, Catholics from Protestant principalities, and Anabaptists were mistreated by everyone.

But ought we now to topple the statue of Johann Philipp because he created a partial peace for some people which brought much suffering to others?

Let me proceed to Johann Philipp's nephew Lothar Franz Schönborn, archbishop of Mainz and bishop of Bamberg at the height of the Baroque era. Lothar Franz was also a politician of peace, a close friend of the Protestant

philosopher and mathematician Leibniz, and a brilliant strategist who became the chief architect of his family's great flowering. As a result of his efforts, one of his nephews, Friedrich Karl, became imperial vice chancellor and built the gigantic Baroque palace of Schönborn outside Vienna. For his services to the imperial house, the emperor gave him an unimaginably huge estate of 148,000 acres in what is today Ukraine. (It remained in the family until 1945, when Soviet troops expropriated it.)

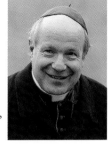

Cardinal Schönborn

## Someday, people will ask: Why didn't you see that within three generations you consumed all the petroleum that took millions of years to create?

Yet as bishops, these Baroque princes were also incredibly active pastors. After serving twenty-nine years as imperial vice chancellor, Friedrich Karl likewise became bishop of Würzburg. During his administration, 156 churches were either newly constructed or renovated. He was able to keep his province out of war and made possible a period of unheard-of prosperity. In his personal life, he was a model of piety.

And so I wonder: Where are the blind spots of our era? Someday, people will ask: Why didn't you see that within three generations you consumed all the petroleum that took millions of years to create? Why didn't you foresee the terrible consequences for humankind of the destruction of the world's

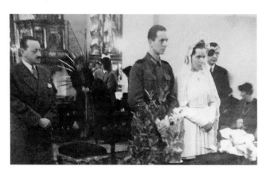

great forests? The difficulty is that we stand in a concrete moment in history and are unable to act as if it were two hundred years later.

**You also inherited difficulties in your immediate family. You father, a courageous opponent of National Socialism, later divorced your mother. How do you deal with your parents' failings?**

When my parents married during World War II, society had already undergone a drastic change following the fall of the European monarchies in 1918. However, their marriage was still socially problematic because my father came from the high nobility and my mother from the lower aristocracy – and besides that, she had a Jewish grandfather.

My parents met during the war; my father was serving on the front. They barely knew each other and never had time to build a life together – I think he simply wanted to have someone at home. In 1944, toward the end of the war, my father deserted to the English and then returned to Germany with the British army. He and my mother didn't find each other again until after the war. It doesn't surprise me that their marriage didn't work out.

So although I was brought up in a deeply Catholic home, I had to learn early on that life sometimes plays out in less-than-ideal ways. Dealing with failure is one of the most important themes of history: one's own personal and family history as well as the history of all

humankind. According to the first pages of the Bible, human history began with a disaster! And that story continues. But I also sensed early on that this drama of imperfection is not the last word. I often heard my mother say, "God writes straight on crooked lines."

**Why is it important to you to know your identity as belonging to a particular family?**

Despite my parents' divorce, the family has been a real home for me, and I think for my siblings as well. That's because family is more than just the parents. We were lucky to have a large extended family. What does "belonging to a family" mean? One of the greatest afflictions of our child-poor society is the lack of family networks. Loneliness can be oppressive if no family is to be found. Surprisingly enough, even in a damaged condition the family is a survival network. The family is not an ideal, yet there is nothing better. The family is affected by our sins and failings. At the same time, it is the place where we are at home and learn our first lessons in socialization. You can see it even in a refugee family like ours, with no permanent home and forced to live in many places during the first postwar years.

**You were still quite young when you felt called to a celibate life. Today, do you miss having children of your own – biological heirs?**

For me, the choice was clear: I was called to become a priest. In the Roman Catholic tradition, that meant forgoing a family of my own, but not forgoing my extended family – I have fifteen grandnieces and nephews.

One question does concern me personally: Would I have been a more mature person had I married and had children? Yet I can also say that I have had a very intense life up to now, with many marvelous encounters and the availability to help others.

There is a reason the celibate life exists and there is a model for it: the life of Jesus. I often ask him, "How did you live your life? You were a strong man" – one can sense that – "and you were a real man! You had marvelous interactions with women. You loved children; they were strongly attracted to you. But you had no wife, no children of your own. How did you manage that?" As yet, I haven't had a clear answer from him. I also ask him: "You were a man with a man's sexuality. How did you live with that?" And he did live with it.

There's one thing you cannot say about Jesus, namely, that he was incapable of forming relationships. The Gospels are witness to wonderful encounters: "Woman, why do you weep?" – his first words upon rising from the dead addressed to Mary Magdalene. And his words to the widow of Nain with her dead son, her only son. What compassion! Jesus was and is a man with a wonderful capacity to relate to others.

**Do you have spiritual heirs? Are there people who have worked with you or been your students and who are a sort of spiritual children?**

I experienced that feeling very strongly with my students when I was a professor. I loved working with them and watching them develop. It was wonderful! There were always people I accompanied as a spiritual director, some of them throught the course of many years. And there are marvelous spiritual friendships. That is something very precious indeed.

Still, I have to admit: when I hear a newly minted grandfather talk with shining eyes about the first time he held his newborn grandchild – that is something I will never experience.

**It's a paradox: today, interest in heredity and genealogy is booming – it has even given rise to an internet industry worth billions of dollars. Modern people, it seems, long for a sense of identity. Yet this is at odds with a** central dogma of modern liberalism: that we can each invent ourselves just as we like.

A tree cannot stand without its roots, and neither can a human being. I often ask young people if they know the names of their great-grandparents, and what they were like. In my father's family, we have a family tree that reaches back into the thirteenth century; on

> To atone and ask forgiveness, the healing of memory, is a real task. The demons of hatred, pride, and nationalism must be banished.

my mother's side, it's only into the seventeenth. I admire Jewish families who can say they are from the tribe of Levi. That's three thousand years of genealogy!

The science of genetics has given us something simple to consider: all of us carry our ancestors in our bodies. They are all there. My genetic code is the inheritance of all my ancestors. And we carry within us an eternal soul that is not the product of our parents, not the product of our genealogy, but God's creation. I am a human being, interwoven with the universe, the cosmos, and all human history. And yet, I am unmistakably unique, an individual created by God.

**What, if anything, do we owe our ancestors?**

We owe our genetic inheritance to them. I carry within me my maternal grandfather's colorblindness, inherited according to Mendelian laws. Do we also carry within us the guilt of our ancestors? There is no such thing as collective guilt, genealogical guilt. But there is a sense in which we are entangled in a history of guilt. My mother always told us that our inherited estate in Bohemia, which was very

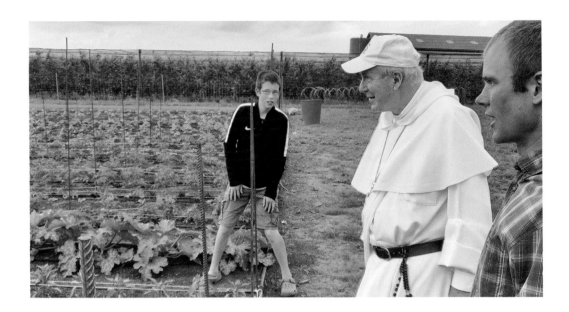

large, came to our family as a result of the Battle of White Mountain in 1620, in which the Bohemian nobility was defeated and partially wiped out. The Holy Roman Emperor rewarded the loyal victors with Bohemian estates. Three centuries later, my family's expulsion from Bohemia after World War II was the endpoint of this painful history.

Even if I don't believe there is such a thing as inherited guilt, we can still assume responsibility for our ancestors' guilt. We assume it precisely because of our faith – by admitting that yes, our ancestors sinned. And we can atone for it and ask for forgiveness. Such paths of healing are important. The Czechs attempted to do just that with the Germans expelled in 1945. To atone and ask forgiveness, the healing of memory, is a real task. The demons of hatred, pride, and nationalism must be banished.

**How does that apply to Christians and the Christian church, especially in overcoming our history of hatred and schism?**

Once, at an ecumenical reception, I remarked that perhaps much of our ecumenical reconciliation within Christianity has to do with the fact that we were deprived of our power. No longer are we the seventeenth-century Protestant and Catholic states that went to war with each other, nor does the pope rule over an ecclesiastical state that wages wars. We live in secular countries. As far as issues of power are concerned, we are marginalized, which is probably also a blessing.

We must remember that Christians have often been persecuted, and still are today. It's interesting that historically our opponents made no distinctions among the various confessions. Christians helped one another in the concentration camps and the gulag; they were all simply Christians. We had to become powerless to surrender ourselves to Christ's power and put our trust in him – not in weaponry, not in political power, but "in demonstration of the Spirit and of power," as Paul says (1 Cor. 2). The lovely thing is that we recognize one another anew, not from the standpoint of our confessions, but with a view to Christ. Whenever I encounter a brother or sister and I see that they really love the

Lord, then there is an immediate basis for communication.

Of course, there are still enormous differences between confessions – in how we worship, for instance – but we know that the center is the same, the center is Christ. As Pope Benedict XVI told us, "What is meant by ecumenism? Simply this: that we listen to one another and learn from one another what it means to be a Christian today." We experience that concretely when I encounter my dear friends in the Bruderhof community and how you live your Christianity! I've learned much from that.

**As a Bruderhof member who moved to Austria last year, I've experienced firsthand this practical work for reconciliation – not least, through your welcome and support as we start a Bruderhof community here. What does this founding of a new Austrian Bruderhof mean to you?**

It is a concrete example of the healing process, since of course the Anabaptist movement, to which the Bruderhof belongs, began here in Austria and neighboring countries five hundred years ago. When Bruderhof members visit the sites of the original Anabaptist communities in Moravia, it inevitably reminds us of how the Anabaptists were driven from their homes under the Holy Roman Empress Maria Theresa. One might say that this expulsion simply reflected the politics of that time. But it also reflected a particular idea of how Christianity and the state should work together. There is a lesson here for us today.

And even now, although we as Catholics and Anabaptists can relate to one another so easily, that doesn't mean that we've already done everything necessary. We must remember our history; we must talk about it with one another. How do you remember, and how do we? What wounds are still open? What

burdens from the past still encumber us? That is the healing of memory that we must carry out simply by talking about our history. But the work of healing itself is the work of the Lord.

**You've spoken often of your concern about the demographic trends in Europe toward a "childless or child-poor society." What hope do you have for the future of the family?**

Every child who is born brings hope. I believe that in his marvelous plan of creation and the creation of man and woman, the Creator gave us a clear sign of the path to follow, whatever course society may take. There were and still are all sorts of experiments like the ones

---

## We carry within us an eternal soul that is not the product of our parents, nor the product of our genealogy, but God's creation.

---

undertaken by the Soviets, who separated children from their parents at an early age. But a young man falls in love with a young woman. They begin life's journey together, get married, and have children. The family is a wonderful network, stronger than any other. I have the greatest confidence in the Creator. We disturbed and abused creation through our sins, and that made a Savior necessary. And God sent us a Savior! Thank the Lord! The Creator laid out the basic pattern, and even after the Fall, he was always there. That is why I simply cannot be pessimistic about the future of the family. ⤳

---

*This interview from September 12, 2020, has been edited for clarity and concision. Translation by David Dollenmayer.*

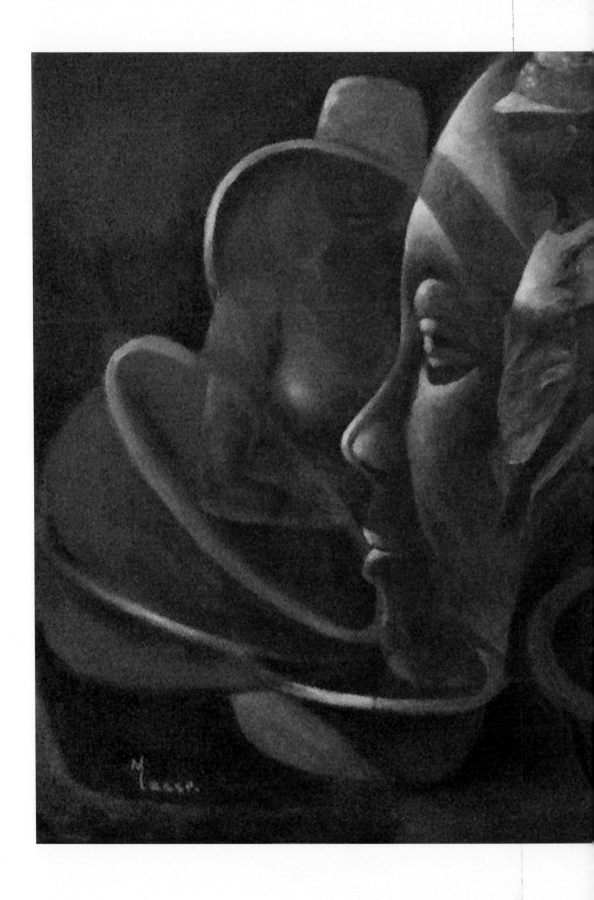

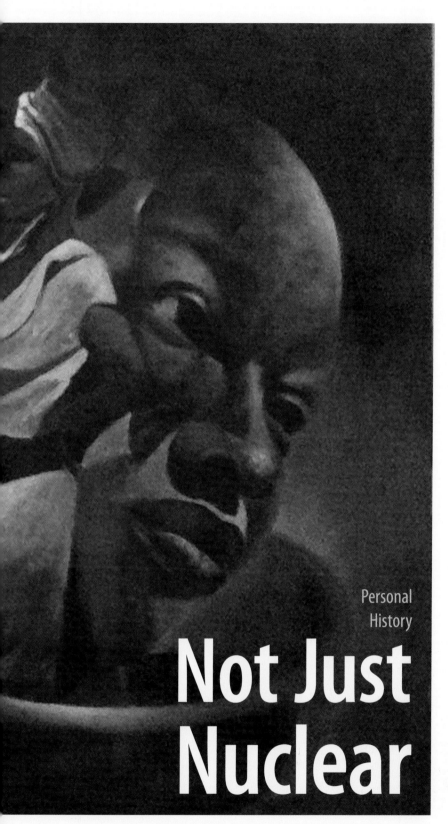

Personal
History

# Not Just Nuclear

Families are
elders long
buried and
generations
yet unborn.

**Edwidge
Danticat**

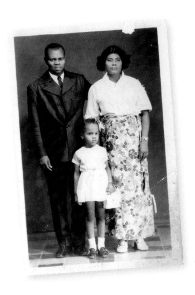

*Above:* The author in 1973, age four, with the uncle and aunt who raised her

*Previous spread:* Massé Mansour, *Untitled,* acrylic, 2017

**S**OMETIMES I THINK my mother and father are parenting me from the grave. A few weeks ago, I dreamt that I was pushing a mini-hatchback up a steep hill, with my mom and dad on either side of me, helping. In the dream, both my parents are the ages they were when they died: my father sixty-nine and my mother eighty-four years old. After Sisyphean effort was exerted toward getting the car to the top of the hill, the three of us celebrated by contemplating the magnificent view of a beautiful green meadow below.

It was close to the sixth anniversary of my mother's death and I often found myself grieving for her in my dreams. The Sisyphean twist, though, was new. Though Sisyphus, the dishonorable king of Corinth, twice cheated death, it turned out that he couldn't cheat life. The punishment for all his murdering and angering the gods was being condemned, day after day, to roll a boulder up a hill, only to have it constantly roll down again.

The day after I had this dream, my seventy-eight-year-old uncle, my father's younger brother, wandered out of his house in the early morning hours, alone and bewildered. A neighbor spotted him and alerted my cousin, his daughter. Suddenly – perhaps not so suddenly – he was living, it seemed, the same day over and over again. My uncle's past and present seemed to have merged. The future was blurred, or had possibly faded altogether. An entire segment of our family history, of which only he had been the caretaker, was no longer available, to us or to him.

Growing up in a multigenerational Haitian family, I never thought of it as "nuclear." For all the term's other meanings, either relating to atoms or energy generation, or even war, when applied to families it seemed limiting. My parents and uncle agreed. Families, they believed, expand like ripples in a pond. Besides, migration forces you to remake your family as well as yourself. Family is not only made up of your living relatives either. It is elders long buried and generations yet unborn, with stories as bridges, and dreams as potential portals.

The idea of my parents communicating from a great distance is not new to me. When my mother and father moved to the United States from Haiti in the 1970s, both to escape a brutal dictatorship and to look for work, they left me and my younger brother behind, in the care of another uncle and his wife. From the time I was four till I was twelve, my parents and I communicated via letters, a weekly phone

*Edwidge Danticat is the author of many books, including, most recently,* Everything Inside: Stories *(Knopf, 2019).*

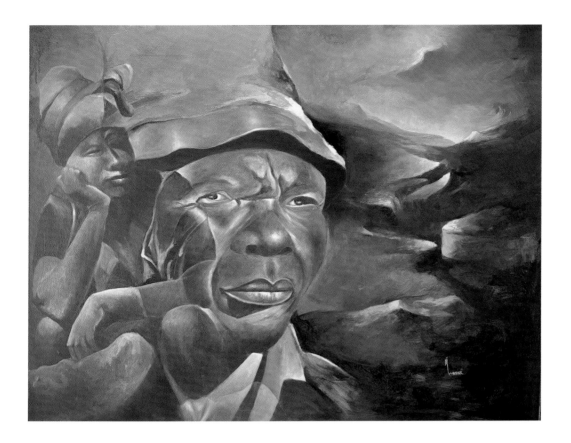

call, and cassette tapes carried by friends and acquaintances between Brooklyn and Port-au-Prince. I was one of half a dozen children whom my aunt and uncle cared for while our parents were working in other countries. This is what family was supposed to do, to help with things you couldn't always do on your own, including raising your children. This is what many families are still doing: while mothers and fathers are incarcerated, or held in immigration detention centers, or fighting opioid or other addictions, family members fill the gap.

Family, as my now-silenced uncle used to say, is whoever is left when everyone else is gone. It is whoever is cleaning up at the end of the party or the funeral repast. It is that person whose one nod might comfort you more than hundreds of words from someone else. Family members share and carry your memories with you.

I feel an immeasurable sense of loss when I think of how family members are disappearing from my uncle's mind. Day by day he has fewer and fewer faces left on which to project his lifetime of memories. I keep wondering if he dreams, and what he might be dreaming about. His own dead parents and siblings? His childhood home in the mountains of southern Haiti? His years spent as a factory worker, cab driver, and car-service owner in New York City? His five sons and daughters? The Bible verses he has recited throughout his life? The final years he'd imagined as a proud grandfather embraced by a large brood of grandchildren, possibly even great-grandchildren?

Perhaps his dreams are vivid, like movies of his own making, but he's probably also experienced hallucinations and night terrors. Like a lot of dementia patients, he might also be

Massé Mansour, *Uncertainties,* acrylic, 2017

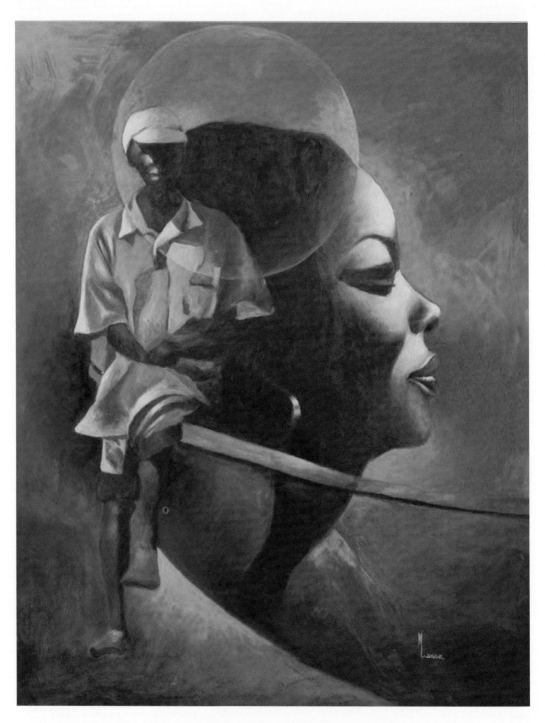

Massé Mansour, *Maternal Longing*, acrylic, 2018

suffering from sundowning, evening agitation and restlessness, when familiar shadows grow mysterious. Could he be confused at sunrising, too, driven by dreams into the street, at dawn? To speak of "sundowning" and "sunrising," though, assigns him much more agency than he appears to have, as if he were Phaethon, dragging the sun behind him across the sky.

When my parents were dying – my father of pulmonary fibrosis and my mother of ovarian cancer – it was their bodies that failed them. During their final days, they were both able to communicate and get plenty off their chests, as they liked to say. My mother might call a loved one and settle a dispute, explain, or apologize. My father would reminisce or advise, telling long stories from which he hoped my brothers and I would learn important lessons, to pass on to our children and they to theirs.

One of my father's stories was about knowing when to leave. When my father was a young man in Haiti, he worked in a shoe store often frequented by the henchmen of the dictatorship. These paramilitary men, the *tonton macoutes*, would walk into the store, grab the best shoes off the shelf, and walk away, and there was nothing either my father or his boss could do about it. My father got a knot in his stomach whenever one of these men walked in, fearing that one day he might feel compelled to resist and get shot. That's when he decided he not only had to leave his job at the shoe store, but leave Haiti in order for his family to have a more stable and peaceful life.

One of my mother's stories was about regrets. After my mother left my younger brother and me in Haiti, she constantly felt like a terrible mother who had abandoned her children. Eventually though, she felt she was mothering us from afar. Whenever she was eating, she told me, she wondered whether we were eating. Whenever she was about to

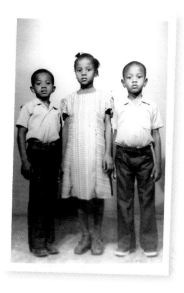

The author, age eight, with her brother and cousin

go to sleep, she asked herself where and how we were going to sleep. She marked her days by our imagined routines, syncing them as much as possible with hers. The only thing that sustained her throughout our eight years apart was her dream of being reunited with us some day. This was one of the reasons both she and my father worked two jobs each, at times, to make our lives and the lives of our two US-born brothers a lot easier than theirs had ever been.

My uncle might no longer recall his early struggle days. He might no longer remember his fear of snow, or his many slips and falls on black ice. He might not fully remember the births of his children or the death of his wife.

Family legacies, my father used to say, are not only about traditions and values passed on from generation to generation. They are also about the actions we take or choose not to take. In the mountain village where my uncle and father were born, a single deed could mark or stain your family's reputation for generations, placing you in a hierarchy that, if only enforced by gossip or shame, might still decide the fate of your progeny. I am not sure that's still true, but my father held on to that notion until his death, in part because it was taught to him by his father, who had learned it from his father. This is why they had to leave the ancestral village and move to the capital, my father would say. Though neither he nor his siblings had committed shameful acts, they longed to start over in a new place where the generational burden was less weighty. Their new beginning was meant to be a reboot, though, not an erasure.

**Family legacies, my father used to say, are about the actions we take or choose not to take. Family legacies are not only about traditions passed on from generation to generation.**

In the midst of all types of losses, our family has come to experience our most painful moments as opportunities to celebrate as well as to mourn. One of my most gut-wrenching memories with my uncle is of seeing him soon after his wife died giving birth to his youngest daughter. Though he was heartbroken, he also looked relieved that out of that terrible tragedy had emerged a beautiful little girl.

When he was finally allowed to bring his daughter home, my parents and I went to visit them. My tiny infant cousin was curled up in her crib, sucking her index and middle finger intently as though she were nursing. My parents and I looked down at her in amazement. She looked so fragile that we were afraid to pick her up.

"Go ahead," my uncle told me, as if reading my thoughts. "She's not going to break. She has life in her."

In Haitian Creole, he said, *"Li gen la vi nan li,"* which he also meant in a spiritual sense. *There is life in her*, not something we were necessarily taking for granted. My uncle might also have said, "She has come a long way to be here. She has traveled very far to reach us."

I picked up my baby cousin and held her close. Her eyes kept fluttering as she half giggled and smiled. My uncle was right. There was plenty of life, and spirit, in her. She had been at that intangible crossroads where she entered this world as her mother abruptly exited. She was filled with both joy and pain.

In Aztec mythology, women who die during childbirth are considered fallen warriors. These women are also believed to travel with the sun throughout the latter part of the day, settling into sundown. My baby cousin's sunrise was filled with stories of battles and triumph. Though her presence was also an absence, she represented as much what we had gained as lost. And my uncle had been there to witness it all.

That night, holding his daughter, my uncle told us he felt as though he had gone into the jaws of hell and yanked her out. It was something that he was also willing to do over and over again if needed, he said.

Perhaps this is what my parents were trying to tell me in that dream the night before my uncle left his house that morning, at dawn. Maybe my parents were reminding me that they too, like my uncle, will always be with me, even when bodies and minds are beyond reach. These days, I have no choice but to hold on to all of them with all my might. That is, after all, what families do. ⬎

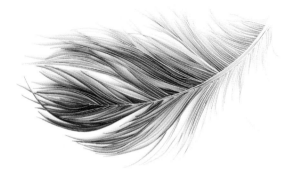

# Dependence

## *Toward an Illiberalism of the Weak*

**LEAH LIBRESCO SARGEANT**

No man or woman is an island, and no one should aspire to be one, either. That, at the core, is the claim of illiberalism, post-liberalism, or any of the other names given to the movement that pushes back against individualism as an ideal. The liberalism of Locke, deeply woven into American culture and political philosophy, takes the individual as the basic unit of society, while an illiberal view looks to traditions, family, and other institutions whose demands define who we are.

It always confuses me that illiberalism is taken as a belligerent ideology – both by its detractors and some of its proponents – as though it were rooted in strength and prepared to wield that power against others. It is contemporary liberalism that begins from an anthropology of independence, and presumes a strength and self-ownership we do not in fact possess.

The best corrective the growing illiberal enthusiasm can offer is not a rival strength – no fist clenched around a flagpole of any standard. Instead it must offer a re-appreciation of weakness – the kind I see in the chubby, fumbling fingers of my daughter, reaching out to her parents.

Yulia Brodskaya, *Feather,* paper quilling

---

*Leah Libresco Sargeant is the author of* Arriving at Amen *(Ave Maria Press, 2015) and* Building the Benedict Option: A Guide to Gathering Two or Three Together in His Name *(Ignatius Press, 2018).*

Yulia Brodskaya, *Coins*, paper quilling

The liberal theory of the independent individual as the basic unit of society is full of exceptions. When my own baby was awaiting birth, paddling away at my insides to strengthen her lungs and her bones, she was decidedly non-autonomous. She is swept out of moral consideration with the claim that she is not a person until she can survive without my involvement.

Of course, after birth, she gained some abilities, but far fewer than she would need to feed herself (much less navigate the free market). But here, the liberal order is a little more generous. Her infancy, her toddlerhood, her childhood is a rounding error – just a brief, aberrant state before she is enumerated among the radically free.

Old age is dismissed similarly. When the aged reach a certain point of weakness and inability, some doctors and ethicists are as ready to deny personhood at the end of life as they were at the beginning. And the end of life is, once again, graciously excused as an exceptional time – there was a lot of autonomy in the middle, so the end can't be held against the individual, or the theory.

All of this is nonsense. It would be fairer to say that dependence is our default state, and self-sufficiency the aberration. Our lives begin and (frequently) end in states of near total dependence, and much of the middle is marked by periods of need.

THIS SHOULDN'T COME as a surprise to the Christian. Even when we are most distant from our dependence on other created beings, we are still dependent on God, who conserves us in being from moment to moment. In a sermon titled "Remembrance of Past Mercies" from Saint John Henry Newman's collection of "Parochial and Plain Sermons," he points out that we are triply dependent on God:

We cannot be our own masters. We are God's property by creation, by redemption, by regeneration. He has a triple claim upon us. Is it not our happiness thus to view the matter? Is it any happiness, or any comfort, to consider that we are our own? It may be thought so by the young and prosperous. . . . But as time goes on, they, as all men, will find that independence was not made for man – that it is an unnatural state – [that] may do for a while, but will not carry us on safely to the end. No, we are creatures; and, as being such, we have two duties, to be resigned and to be thankful.

A world that holds up independence as the ideal offers us two rival duties: to obscure our dependence and to be resentful of it. No woman can lightly assent to the illusion of autonomy. Because a baby is alien to the world of self-ownership, every woman's citizenship in that imaginary republic is tenuous. A world of autonomous individuals can't acknowledge both woman and child simultaneously. The sheer amount of work it takes to stifle fertility, put eggs on ice, or pump milk for a baby not welcome outside the home makes it clear that there is something untruthful and sharp-clawed at loose in the world.

Fear and hatred of weakness and dependence wound the dependent most obviously, but are poison to all, even the people who are strong at present. Without repeated reminders that the broken are beloved, how can we remember who God is?

Our physical weakness is a training ground for our struggles with moral weakness. There is no physical infirmity we can endure that is more humiliating than our susceptibility to sin. The elderly woman with tremors that leave her unable to lift her cup to her lip is not, in the final sense, weaker than any vigorous young man who finds he must echo Paul and admit, "For I do not do the good I want, but the evil I

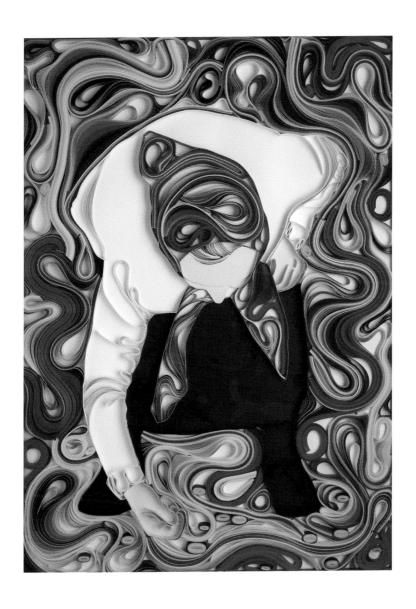

It would be fairer to say that
dependence is our default
state, and self-sufficiency
the aberration.

do not want is what I do" (Rom. 7:19).

There is a blessing in the inescapability of physical weakness that breaks our pride. Sister Teresa de Cartagena, a fifteenth-century Cistercian nun from Spain, wrote *Arboleda de los enfermos* (*Grove of the Infirm*) as a spiritual reflection on her own deafness. Sister Teresa writes: "Divine generosity invites all to this blessed feast, but suffering grabs the infirm by their cloak and makes them enter by force."

She interprets Christ's parable of the great banquet, in which, she says, "the infirm are brought by force to the magnificent feast of eternal health, because their suffering grabs them by the cloak and makes them enter through the door of good works; for if we do not enter through that door, we will not be able to reach the greatest heights of honor, which is to be seated at the table of divine generosity. O blessed convent of the infirm!"

So long as we are not currently weak in body, we are tempted to view ourselves as whole. In the absence of visible blemish, we blunt our longing to become whole. And, lest we be tempted to consider the truth, we need only look at how far from us we have pushed those who are weak. We imagine that we can't possibly be discardable, like they are, and therefore our souls must be unspotted.

A society that cannot imagine placing the weak at its center, that forgets that society exists for the weak, will be drawn towards the Manichaean modes of cancel culture. We see sin but not grace – we try to find and throw out the bad apples, whom (we think) no one can restore to righteousness. Or we see ourselves mirrored in the most notorious sinners, and work to deny sin, since we don't want to be cast out with them.

Paul points us towards the proper expression of our vulnerability in his second letter to the Corinthians. He struggles with his own thorn, and asks the Lord to spare him. "Three times I appealed to the Lord about this, that it would leave me, but he said to me, 'My grace is sufficient for you, for power is made perfect in weakness.' So, I will boast all the more gladly of my weaknesses, so that the power of Christ may dwell in me" (2 Cor. 12:8–9).

To give an honest accounting of ourselves, we must begin with our weakness and fragility. We cannot structure our politics or our society to serve a totally independent, autonomous person who never has and never will exist. Repeating that lie will leave us bereft: first, of sympathy from our friends when our physical weakness breaks the implicit promise that no one can keep, and second, of hope, when our moral weakness should lead us, like the prodigal, to rush back into the arms of the Father who remains faithful. Our present politics can only be challenged by an illiberalism that cherishes the weak and centers its policies on their needs and dignity.

> We cannot structure our politics or our society to serve a totally independent, autonomous person who never has and never will exist.

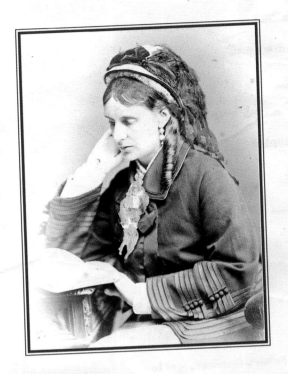

# THE PRAYING FEMINIST

## Josephine Butler,

**A Pioneer of First Wave Feminism, Sacrificed her Respectability to Fight for Prostitutes — Because of her Christian Faith.**

### SARAH C. WILLIAMS

I**N 1927 MILLICENT FAWCETT**, leader of the British suffragist movement, called Josephine Butler "the most distinguished woman of the nineteenth century."[1] Among the first feminist activists, Butler had raised public awareness of the plight of destitute women, worked to address human trafficking, and led a vigorous campaign to secure equal rights for women.

Over the last two years I have been studying this woman's life, and I have been deeply impacted by her faith. Josephine Butler (1828–1908) lived a life immersed in prayer. Prayer emerges in her writing as an intimate dialogue with Christ but also as the pivotal dynamic in a radical social and political vision. It was in prayer that Butler reimagined her world and enabled others to do the same. Crucially, it was in prayer that Butler reimagined the figure of the prostitute – the object of fear, hatred, and

1. M. G. Fawcett and E. M. Turner, *Josephine Butler: Her Work's and Principles and Their Meaning for the Twentieth Century* (London: Association for Moral and Social Hygiene, 1927), 1.

*Dr. Sarah C. Williams has taught history at Oxford and Regent College. She lives with her husband, Paul, in Burford, England. Sarah is the author of* Perfectly Human: Nine Months with Cerian *(Plough, 2018).*

lust – as a human being with dignity, voice, and equal worth before the law.

As a child, Josephine's imagination was captured by Christ as she listened to the Bible read aloud in her home. Her father, John Grey of Dilston, was an important landowner in Northumberland and, in keeping with tradition, the family attended the local Anglican church. But as a teen Josephine was drawn to lively evening gatherings at a small Methodist church. She traveled to these meetings with a servant in the Dilston household, the two of them riding in the back of a cart, sitting on piles of sacking. It was during these years that she developed a lifelong habit of prayer. Reflecting back on this period Butler writes:

> I spoke to Him in solitude as a person who could answer. I sometimes gave whole nights to prayer, because the day was not sufficiently my own. Do not imagine that on these occasions I worked myself up into any excitement: there was much pain in such an effort, and dogged determination required, nor was it devotional sentiment which urged me on. It was a desire to know God and my relation to Him.[2]

IN 1852 JOSEPHINE MARRIED George Butler, a classics tutor at Oxford University. When Josephine first arrived at Oxford she was delighted by the place. Coming from a wealthy and liberal-minded family, she was no stranger to learning. But, when a highly controversial novel appeared in the bookshops, Josephine's delight in the culture of Oxford gave way to disillusionment. Written in 1853 by Elizabeth Gaskell, *Ruth* told the story of a young woman seduced by a wealthy gentleman, abandoned by her lover, pregnant, thrown from her workplace without a reference, shunned by her family and by

society. Butler was captivated by the story. At the next Oxford dinner party, she sat in stunned silence listening to the learned men of the city scorn the book. There, around the table, Butler saw displayed the same attitudes she had read about in the novel. During the same period of time, Butler also began to meet young women on the streets of Oxford, some of

> "I spoke to Him in solitude as a person who could answer. I sometimes gave whole nights to prayer, because the day was not sufficiently my own."

them little more than children, who had been brought to the city to feed the sexual appetites of the male establishment. For the first time in her life, Butler encountered the underworld of Victorian prostitution.

The plight of one woman in particular haunted Butler. Barely eighteen and left to face a pregnancy alone, in her distress she killed her infant at birth. The scandalous case of infanticide was reported in the press; the woman was depicted as the essence of sin and thrown into prison at hard labor. Butler also saw the crime which was never spoken of: the infant's father sitting at a dinner party pontificating about Gaskell's novel before going on his regular visit to the other side of town. The public face and the private life, protected by the safe wall of male privilege!

When the same woman was released from prison, the Butlers brought her to live in their home right in the middle of Oxford. It was

2. Butler to Professor Benjamin Jowett, n.d. (ca. 1860–70), Josephine Butler Collection, The Women's Library.

a public participation in this woman's pain, and an indictment. The doors of Oxford closed on the Butlers and the couple found themselves on the other side of a wall of prejudice.

Years later, now forty-two and a busy headmaster's wife and homemaker, Josephine Butler found herself on a damp stone floor in a large cellar under the Brownlow workhouse in the port of Liverpool. The family had moved to Liverpool from Cheltenham, where George Butler worked as a schoolteacher after leaving his position at Oxford. The bare cellar was an "oakum shed." Here, in exchange for bread and a few nights' shelter, women, most of them otherwise engaged in penny prostitution, separated the loose fibers of old rope to be used for caulking wooden ships. "I went down to the oakum sheds," Butler writes, "and begged admission."

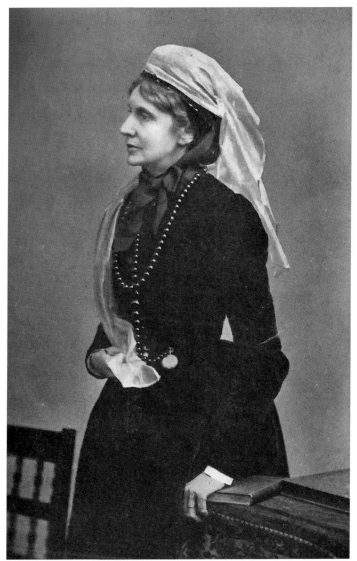

> I was taken into an immense gloomy vault filled with women and girls – more than two hundred probably at that time. I sat on the floor among them and picked oakum. They laughed at me and told me my fingers were of no use for that work, which was true. But while they laughed we became friends.[3]

In the months following this first visit, Butler taught these Liverpool women to pray. She recalls one of these visits vividly in her memoir:

3. *Josephine E. Butler: An Autobiographical Memoir* (Bristol: J. W. Arrowsmith, 1909), 59.

> I recollect a tall, dark, handsome girl standing up in our midst, among the damp refuse and lumps of tarred rope and repeating . . . the words of Jesus all through ending with, "Peace I leave with you. My peace I give unto you. Let not your hearts be troubled, neither let them be afraid." She had selected it herself, and they listened in perfect silence – this audience, wretched, bedraggled, ignorant, criminal some, and wild and defiant others. . . . I said, "Let us kneel and cry to that same Jesus who spoke these words." And down on their knees they fell every one of them, reverently on that

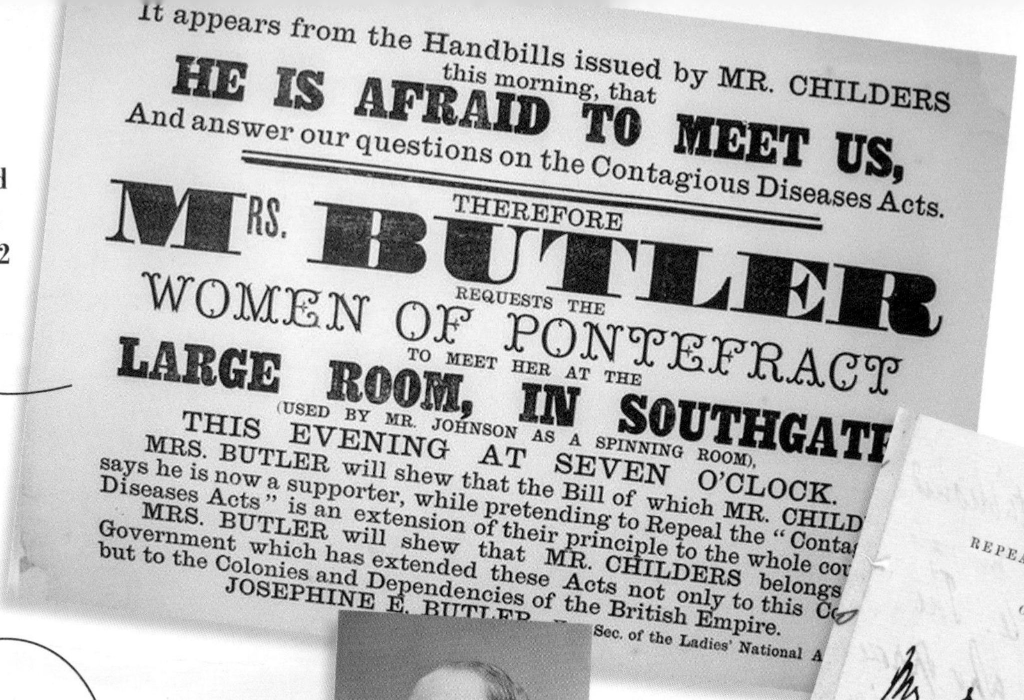

It appears from the Handbills issued by MR. CHILDERS
this morning, that
**HE IS AFRAID TO MEET US,**
And answer our questions on the Contagious Diseases Acts.
THEREFORE
**MRS. BUTLER**
REQUESTS THE
WOMEN OF PONTEFRACT
TO MEET HER AT THE
**LARGE ROOM, IN SOUTHGATE**
(USED BY MR. JOHNSON AS A SPINNING ROOM),
**THIS EVENING AT SEVEN O'CLOCK.**
MRS. BUTLER will shew that the Bill of which MR. CHILDERS
says he is now a supporter, while pretending to Repeal the "Contagious
Diseases Acts" is an extension of their principle to the whole country.
MRS. BUTLER will shew that MR. CHILDERS belongs to a
Government which has extended these Acts not only to this Country,
but to the Colonies and Dependencies of the British Empire.
JOSEPHINE E. BUTLER, Hon. Sec. of the Ladies' National Association.

Handbill issued prior to a talk during the 1872 Pontefract by-election

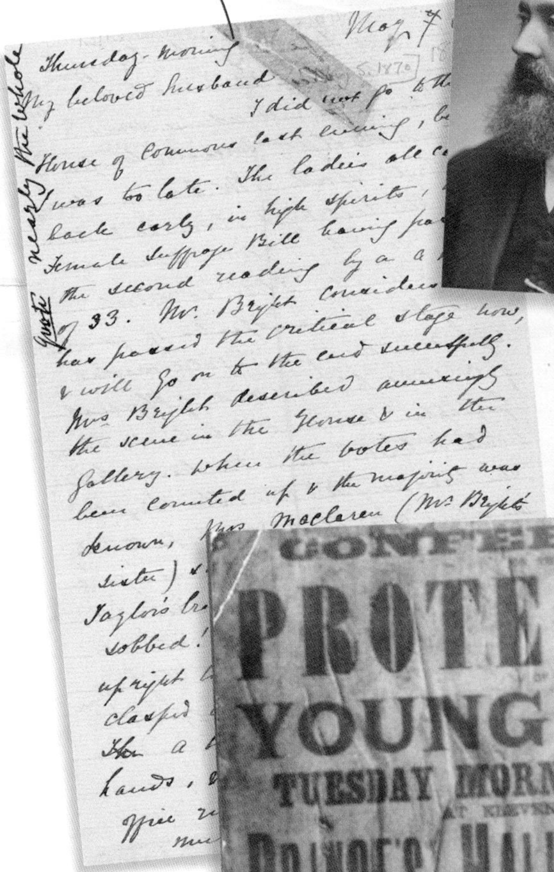

Letter from Josephine Butler to her husband, George, in 1872

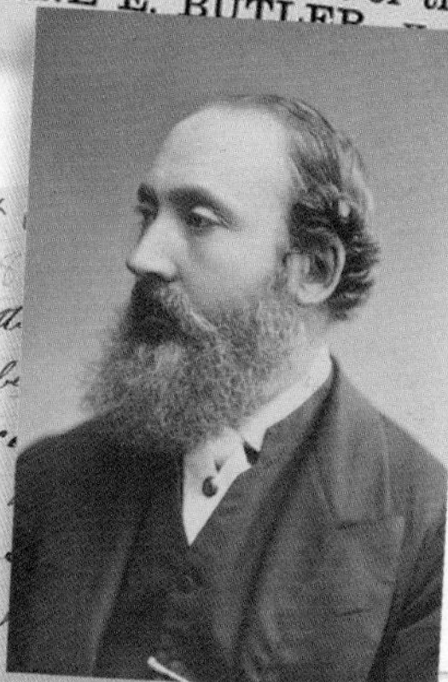

George Butler

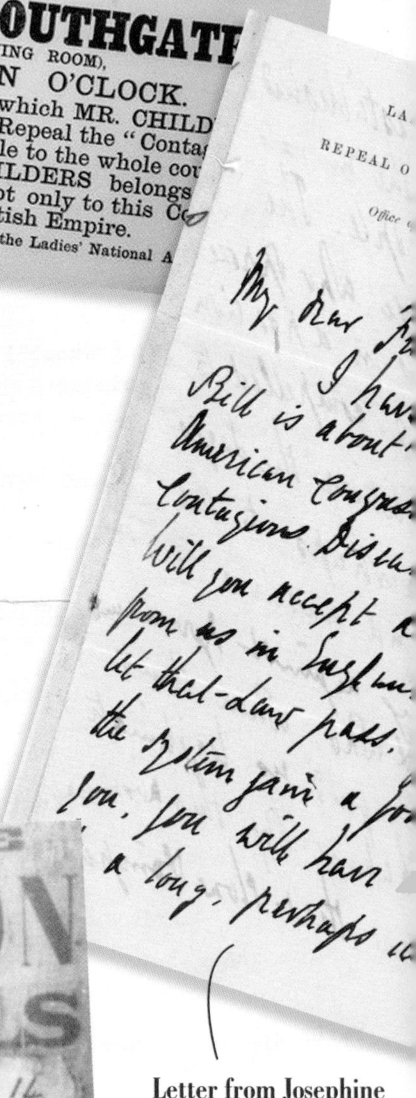

Letter from Josephine Butler to William Lloyd Garrison, an American abolitionist and friend, in 1874, warning against the passing of a bill similar to the Contagious Diseases Act

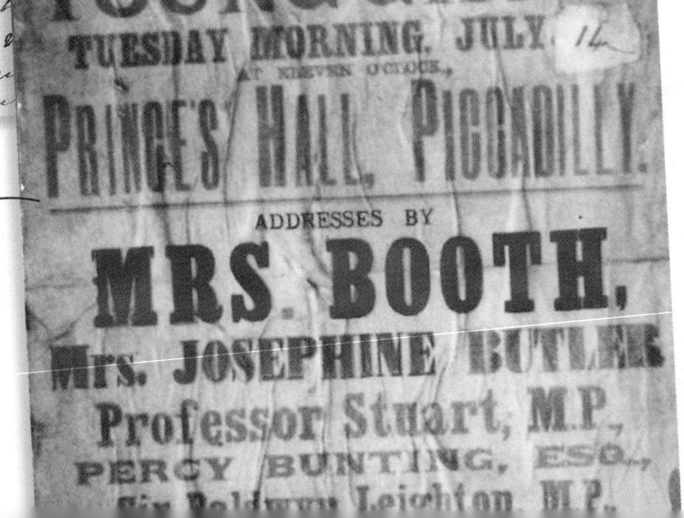

CONFERENCE
PROTECTION
YOUNG GIRLS
TUESDAY MORNING, JULY 14.
AT ELEVEN O'CLOCK,
PRINCE'S HALL, PICCADILLY.
ADDRESSES BY
**MRS. BOOTH,**
Mrs. JOSEPHINE BUTLER,
Professor Stuart, M.P.
PERCY BUNTING, ESQ.,

Poster advertising a conference held by Catherine Booth and Josephine Butler, July 1885, London

damp stone floor, some saying the words after me, others moaning and weeping. It was a strange sound that united wail – continuous, pitiful, strong – like a great sigh or murmur of vague desire and hope, issuing from the heart of despair, piercing the gloom and murky atmosphere of that vaulted room and reaching to the heart of God.[4]

What these women in the oakum shed did not know at the time was the extent of Butler's personal grief at this point in her life. The Butlers had four children, three boys and one girl. Two years before the scene depicted here, in August 1864, the Butlers' daughter, Eva, fell from the banisters in the family home onto the tiled hallway below. Eva died in agony after every attempt to save her failed. "Never can I lose that memory," Butler wrote years later, "the fall, the sudden cry, and then the silence. She was our only daughter, the light and joy of our lives."[5]

For two years after Eva's death, Butler wrestled with depression and despair. It was during this time that she first visited the oakum sheds. "I had no clear idea beyond that," she writes, "no plan for helping others; my sole wish was to plunge into the heart of some human misery and to say (as I then knew I could) to afflicted people, I understand: I too have suffered."[6]

In the mid-nineteenth century there was nothing unusual in middle-class women doing "rescue work" among prostitutes or "fallen women," as they were known. But Butler refused to call her visits to the Brownlow workhouse rescue work; instead, she talked about individual women with names, faces, and histories – women who were her friends. She refused to use the term "prostitute" or "fallen woman" and instead adopted the word "outcast" to describe the lives of these women.

For two years Butler continued to visit her friends. When some of the women became too ill to work, she invited them to live with her family in her home. Later, she set up small houses of rest in which women who had formerly eked out an existence on the streets could find refuge and employment.

In a unique way, Butler connected the experience of personal grief with the corporate grief of womankind. She understood her vocation as an act of intercession in which she entered into the experience of the outcast woman. There is an intrinsic link in Butler's writing between anguish and the facility to perceive and name injustice. Personal pain becomes political pain, which in turn becomes the seedbed for lasting cultural change.

At every point, Butler contrasts the observance of religious codes by pious and respectable people with the desperate cry of the outcast and her simple longing for God. It is the outcast who is heard by God when she prays. Christ, Butler insists, not only welcomes the outcast, he *became* the outcast, submitting to the shame of exclusion in order to overthrow existing categories and definitions of power. God does not preside in judgment but rather enters in, like Butler, as a friend who suffers *with*.

WHILE BUTLER CONTINUED to visit these women in Liverpool, Parliament passed a series of laws known as the Contagious Diseases Acts. Instituted in 1864 and extended in 1867 and 1869, these laws were passed to deal with the

---

4.  Butler, *Autobiographical Memoir*, 60.
5.  Butler, *Autobiographical Memoir*, 49.
6.  Butler, *Autobiographical Memoir*, 58.

rapid spread of venereal disease among the armed forces in Britain. Under the terms of the Acts, any woman residing in a garrison town or port and suspected of prostitution could be detained by the police and subjected to a fortnightly medical examination. If the woman was found to be suffering from venereal disease, she could be kept in a locked hospital unit for a period of up to nine months. At the end of this period, the woman was given a certificate to prove to future male clientele that her body was free from contamination. If a woman refused compulsory examination, she was brought before the magistrate where she bore sole responsibility to prove her virtue.

The Acts were understood as sanitary expedients. It was generally believed that forced examination was the only way to deal with what was an epidemic of venereal disease. But Butler saw these Acts through the eyes of her friends in Liverpool. For her, the Acts were a concrete symbol of an invidious sexual double standard that caused untold suffering and grief. A woman, once compromised sexually, had no way back, and yet society turned a blind eye to men's so-called "natural proclivities."

In 1869 a small Ladies National Association formed to oppose the bill. Butler was asked to lead. Her decision to oppose the Acts caused an outcry among affluent, intellectual women of her own social circle. To take up such a cause was to waste one's talents on a futile and morally dubious enterprise. It was one thing to rescue individual women from lives of prostitution, but quite another to address the systemic issues of sexual injustice.

On January 1, 1870, under Butler's leadership, the Ladies National Association issued a sharply worded eight-point manifesto denouncing the Contagious Diseases Acts as a blatant example of class and sex discrimination. The Acts, it argued, were unconstitutional

and deprived disadvantaged women of their legal rights. To detain an individual without evidence or trial, and to force her to submit to a degrading examination, was a travesty of the rule of law. Moreover, by placing culpability

> If one hoped to reconfigure social and political realities, Butler believed, one had to start with personal prayer.

singularly on women, the Acts sanctioned discrimination. As Butler wrote in an influential 1871 essay: "The danger of the whole community is imminent when the safeguards of law and constitutional right are swept away from any portion of the community."[7] All future reform would be impossible, she argued, while some humans were set aside to be bought and sold as chattel for the purpose of illicit pleasure that was then excused and hidden by polite society, and endorsed by the state.

Butler had issued her challenge. Yet, what seemed self-evidently right to her did not to those who benefited in one way or another from the existing order of things. It took sixteen years of tireless work before the Contagious Diseases Acts were finally removed from the statute books. During this time, Butler was physically assaulted on many occasions. Her family was subject to repeated death threats and several arson attacks. Butler was pelted with excrement when she stood up to speak, and on one occasion it took fourteen bodyguards to protect her from a violent mob

7. Josephine E. Butler, *Social Purity* (London: Morgan and Scott, 1879), 19.

as she moved from a train carriage to address an audience at a town hall.

Throughout the campaign, Butler prayed with women on the streets, and taught others to do the same. She prayed with leaders from every political party and every religious denomination. She formed networks of prayer that connected those who lacked social and political agency with those who held great power. The relational encounters she facilitated between different groups and social classes challenged existing cultural and political categories. Crossing class, educational, and religious divides, the Ladies National Association grew over time into the backbone of an emergent women's movement.

This group worked among registered prostitutes, gathering evidence, hearing testimonies, and collecting statistics. Its members visited working-class families the length and breadth of Britain and, after 1874, across continental Europe. They introduced local educational and employment reforms, gave legal aid where there was none, encouraged women to resist the legal requirements of the Acts, and formed links in Parliament.

If one hoped to reconfigure social and political realities, Butler believed, one had to start with personal prayer. Without being alone with God, individuals would remain immersed in the existing cultural environment, with its prevailing definitions of power: class power, sexual power, and religious power. Without prayer the conscience would become numbed and passion dulled, leaving the individual

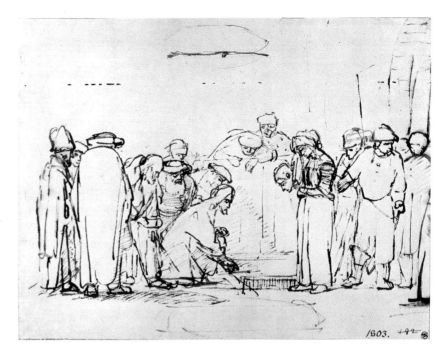

Rembrandt Harmenszoon van Rijn, *Jesus and the Adulteress*

unable to think and act with independent judgment.

Throughout her life, Butler continued to spend a portion of each morning alone in prayer. How will we find the freedom to imagine something new, Butler asked, if we are subject to the noisy tyranny of a society that squeezes us into its way of defining others? The person who prays participates in God's imagination, coming to see as God sees. Those who pray are set free from enculturation and drawn into active agency with God to mobilize and effect deep and lasting change.

This is Josephine Butler's legacy: a fresh social and political imagination. The prostitute – understood by Victorian culture as refuse – became for Butler a sign not only of grief and pain but also of Jesus' identification with the excluded. It was this compassionate identification with others on the margins of society that made Butler's work so transformative and of such lasting significance, inspiring subsequent generations to seek fundamental changes in the ways men and women are treated in society. ⤳

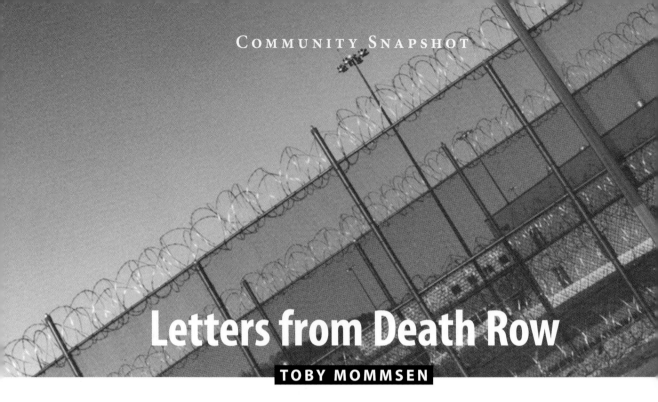

# Letters from Death Row

## TOBY MOMMSEN

### *How Our Family Gained an Incarcerated "Older Brother"*

**H**IS PALMS WERE SPREAD against the thick glass as widely as the handcuffs would allow. His broad smile beamed through; his greeting echoed on the concrete walls. It was a noncontact visit, but nothing could block his joy – nor his fears, hurts, and regrets – in our two hours together.

It was September 14, 1995: my first visit with Tyrone (not his real name) on death row. My first-grade daughter had sent me on the fifty-minute drive from our home to learn why her letter had gone unanswered. Every student in Rose's class had written to someone on the state's register of capital cases. Everyone else got a reply. Why didn't "her prisoner" write back?

Tyrone told me: too many friends on the outside had deserted him. He couldn't risk another heartbreak, he said, least of all with a child befriending him. His own daughter was growing up fatherless. But he promised to stay in touch with our family.

That initial visit to death row twenty-five years ago forged a friendship and launched my family on a surprising journey. "Inmate Mail – Department of Corrections" became a regular in our mailbox.

> Dear Rose,
> Thank you for writing to me again. It is always so nice to get messages in your handwriting. Did your school go on the fall hike yet? When you get back from the hike I want you to tell me about it. Enjoy yourself and learn all you can. You are in my prayers.
> Love, your big brother T

After two years of friendship, I took our oldest son and daughter to visit Tyrone. There were other families and kids in the waiting room. I think the guards must have had kids too; it

---

*Toby Mommsen and his wife, Johanna, live at Platte Clove, a Bruderhof in Elka Park, New York.*

was hard to keep their sense of absolute control with the youngsters around. Concrete and steel are no match for children.

> Dear Toby,
> It was wonderful to get the children's pictures. The kids are just growing and growing. I love to see that.
>
> I should be so very glad that God gives us a chance to redeem ourselves. I want so much to be a better person. Your efforts to forgive me, to stick by me, to love me are not in vain.
>
> Today is one day where I do not feel like a mistake. That is because I love you, brother, and I know you care about me. Please know I am sorry for not being an honest man in the past. Change happens but only through God.

When Tyrone's mother accompanied his young daughter across the state by bus to visit her dad in prison, we hosted them overnight. Our three-month-old son, Sidney, gained a new grandmother, and Rose gained a new friend her own age. For our family, that weekend became one of the highlights of the summer.

One day I got a letter from another inmate on Tyrone's block telling me that Tyrone was bottoming out in depression. But the letters kept coming.

> Dear Toby, Johanna, and family,
> I was never taught how to love, and failed to recognize love when it was given to me. The guilt and shame I feel today is the result of not liking who I am. Please give me the chance to repair the damage I've done to all those I've abused. Please forgive me.

It was five years later that this brief letter shocked us:

> Hello brother. Just a quick note to let you know the Governor signed my execution warrant and set my execution date for October 3. I only can have immediate family visits but I will have someone call you. You can call my lawyer.

> Please know that I love you, Johanna, and each of your children. Keep me in prayer. My lawyers are working very hard. I will write soon.
>
> Love with all my heart, T

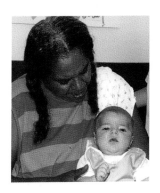

So our friend finally had a date with death. A final square on the calendar. We felt sick; we wrote letters on his behalf. Thankfully, Tyrone received a stay of execution. Then another date was set, and again overturned.

Tyrone is still alive, still behind bars. I have often wished I could share him with other people, help them see and know him. Even those of use who care about Tyrone can fill our minds with wide-ranging ideas and pursue all sorts of interests. We get on with our lives. For him, there's no escape.

*Tyrone's mother holding one of the author's children*

Today, my kids are grown and flown. We still exchange letters with Tyrone and manage an occasional visit. His case moved slowly, but finally, after thirty-two years on death row, a judge threw out his death sentence. At last, visits can include a hug, sitting across a table, sharing a vending-machine snack.

Because of Tyrone, my children have learned to know – just a little – how the world looks and feels from death row. Whatever their ventures in life, they'll bring with them a connection to "big brother T," who has struggled so hard just to stay alive and to stay sane. Who is still struggling.

What has our connection to Tyrone brought to him? A few moments of encouragement, I hope, during the long years of imprisonment, though this is little enough in the face of the cruelties of the system in which he remains trapped. Our lives, in any case, are the richer for knowing this man. ⤳

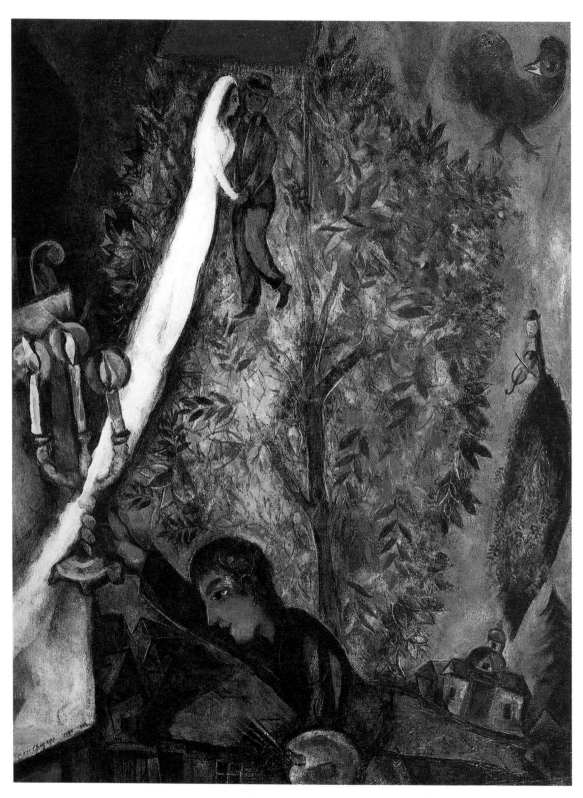

Marc Chagall, *The Tree of Life*, 1948

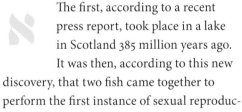

# The Beautiful Institution

*The Story of Marriage in Seven Key Moments*

**RABBI LORD JONATHAN SACKS**

I WANT TO BEGIN by telling the story of the most beautiful idea in the history of civilization: the idea of the love that brings new life into the world. There are of course many ways of telling the story, and this is just one. But to me it is a story of seven key moments, each of them surprising and unexpected.

The first, according to a recent press report, took place in a lake in Scotland 385 million years ago. It was then, according to this new discovery, that two fish came together to perform the first instance of sexual reproduction known to science. Until then all life had propagated itself asexually, by cell division, budding, fragmentation or parthenogenesis, all of which are far simpler and more economical than the division of life into male and female, each with a different role in creating and sustaining life.

When we consider, even in the animal kingdom, how much effort and energy the coming together of male and female takes, in terms of displays, courtship rituals, rivalries, and violence, it is astonishing that sexual reproduction ever happened at all. Biologists are still not quite sure why it did – some say to offer protection against parasites, or immunities against disease. Others say it's simply that the meeting of opposites generates diversity.

---

*Rabbi Lord Jonathan Sacks is an international faith leader, philosopher, theologian, and author, most recently of* Morality: Restoring the Common Good in Divided Times *(Basic Books, 2020). He served as the Chief Rabbi of the United Hebrew Congregations of the Commonwealth from 1991 to 2013.*

But one way or another, the fish in Scotland discovered something new and beautiful that's been copied ever since by virtually all advanced forms of life. Life begins when male and female meet and embrace.

 The second unexpected development was the unique challenge posed to *Homo sapiens* by two factors: we stood upright, which constricted the female pelvis, and we had bigger brains – a 300 percent increase – which meant larger heads. The result was that human babies had to be born more prematurely than any other species, and so needed parental protection for much longer. This made parenting more demanding among humans than any other species, the work of two people rather than one.

Hence the phenomenon, very rare among mammals, of human pair bonding, unlike other species where the male contribution tends to end with the act of impregnation. Among most primates, fathers don't even recognize their children, let alone care for them. Elsewhere in the animal kingdom motherhood is almost universal but fatherhood is rare. So what emerged along with the human person was the union of the biological mother and father to care for their child. Thus far nature, but then came culture, and the third surprise.

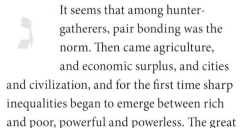

**From monogamy the rich and powerful lose and the poor and powerless gain.**

It seems that among hunter-gatherers, pair bonding was the norm. Then came agriculture, and economic surplus, and cities and civilization, and for the first time sharp inequalities began to emerge between rich and poor, powerful and powerless. The great ziggurats of Mesopotamia and pyramids of ancient Egypt, with their broad bases and narrow tops, were monumental statements in stone of hierarchical societies in which the few had power over the many. And the most obvious expression of power among alpha males, of whatever group, is to dominate access to fertile mates and thus maximize the handing on of genes to the next generation.

Hence polygamy, which exists in 95 percent of mammal species and 75 percent of cultures known to anthropology. Polygamy is the ultimate expression of inequality because it means that many males never get the chance to have a wife and child. And sexual envy has been, throughout history, among animals as well as humans, a prime driver of violence.

That is what makes the first chapter of Genesis so revolutionary with its statement that every human being, regardless of class, color, culture, or creed, is in the image and likeness of God himself. We know that in the ancient world it was rulers, kings, emperors, and pharaohs who were held to be in the image of God. So what Genesis was saying was that we are all royalty. We each have equal dignity in the kingdom of faith under the sovereignty of God.

From this it follows that we each have an equal right to form a marriage and have children, which is why, regardless of how we read the story of Adam and Eve – and there are differences between Jewish and Christian readings – the norm presupposed by that story is: one woman, one man. Or as the Bible itself says: "That is why a man leaves his father and mother and is united to his wife, and they become one flesh."

Monogamy did not immediately become the norm, even within the world of the Bible.

But many of its most famous stories, about the tension between Sarah and Hagar, or Leah and Rachel and their children, or David and Bathsheba, or Solomon's many wives, are all critiques that point the way to monogamy.

And there is a deep connection between monotheism and monogamy, just as there is, in the opposite direction, between idolatry and adultery. Monotheism and monogamy are about the all-embracing relationship between I and Thou, myself and one other, be it a human or the divine Other.

What makes the emergence of monogamy unusual is that it is normally the case that the values of a society are those imposed on it by the ruling class. And the ruling class in any hierarchical society stands to gain from promiscuity and polygamy, both of which multiply the chances of its genes being handed on to the next generation. From monogamy the rich and powerful lose and the poor and powerless gain. So the return of monogamy goes against the normal grain of social change and is a real triumph for the equal dignity of all. Every bride and every groom are royalty, every home a palace when furnished with love.

The fourth remarkable development was the way this transformed moral life. We've all become familiar with the work of evolutionary biologists using computer simulations and the iterated prisoner's dilemma to explain why reciprocal altruism exists among all social animals. We behave to others as we would wish them to behave to us, and we respond to them as they respond to us. As C. S. Lewis pointed out in his book *The Abolition of Man*, reciprocity is the Golden Rule shared by all the great civilizations.

What was new and remarkable in the Hebrew Bible was the idea that *love*, not just fairness, is the driving principle of the moral life. Three loves. "Love the Lord your God with all your heart, all your soul, and all your might." "Love your neighbor as yourself." And, repeated no less than thirty-six times in the Mosaic books, "Love the stranger because you know what it feels like to be a stranger." Or to put it another way: just as God created the natural world in love and forgiveness, so we are charged with creating the social world in love and forgiveness. And that love is a flame lit in marriage and the family. Morality is the love between husband and wife, parent and child, extended outward to the world.

The fifth development shaped the entire structure of Jewish experience. In ancient Israel an originally secular form of agreement, called a covenant, was taken and transformed into a new way of thinking about the relationship between God and humanity, in the case of Noah, and between God and a people in the case of Abraham and later the Israelites at Mount Sinai. A covenant is like a marriage. It is a mutual pledge of loyalty and trust between two or more persons, each respecting the dignity and integrity of the other, to work together to achieve together what neither can achieve alone. And there is one thing even God cannot achieve alone, which is to live within the human heart. That needs us.

So the Hebrew word *emunah*, wrongly translated as faith, really means faithfulness, fidelity, loyalty, steadfastness, not walking away even when the going gets tough, trusting the other and honoring the other's trust in us.

What covenant did, and we see this in almost all the prophets, was to understand the relationship between us and God in terms of the relationship between bride and groom, wife and husband. Love thus became not only the basis of morality but of theology. In Judaism faith is a marriage. Rarely was this more beautifully stated than by Hosea when he said in the name of God:

I will betroth you to me forever;
I will betroth you in righteousness and justice, love and compassion.
I will betroth you in faithfulness, and you will know the Lord.

Jewish men say those words every weekday morning as we wind the strap of our tefillin around our finger like a wedding ring. Each morning we renew our marriage with God.

This led to a sixth and quite subtle idea that truth, beauty, goodness, and life itself do not exist in any one person or entity but in the "between," what Martin Buber called *Das Zwischenmenschliche*, the interpersonal, the counterpoint of speaking and listening, giving and receiving. Throughout the Hebrew Bible and the rabbinic literature, the vehicle of truth is conversation. In revelation God speaks and asks us to listen. In prayer we speak and ask God to listen. There is never only one voice. In the Bible the prophets argue with God. In the Talmud rabbis argue with one another. In fact, I sometimes think the reason God chose the Jewish people was because he loves a good argument. Judaism is a conversation scored for many voices, never more passionately than in the Song of Songs, a duet between a woman and a man, the beloved and her lover, that Rabbi Akiva called the holy of holies of religious literature.

All this led to the seventh outcome, that in Judaism the home and the family became the central setting of the life of faith. In the only verse in the Hebrew Bible to explain why God chose Abraham, he says: "I have known him so that he will instruct his children and his household after him to keep the way of the Lord by doing what is right and just." Abraham was chosen not to rule an empire, command an army, perform miracles, or deliver prophecies, but simply to be a parent.

In one of the most famous lines in Judaism, which we say every day and night, Moses commands, "You shall teach these things repeatedly to your children, speaking of them when you sit in your house or when you walk on the way, when you lie down and when you rise up." Parents are to be educators, education is the conversation between the generations, and the first school is the home.

So JEWS BECAME an intensely family-oriented people, and it was this that saved us from tragedy. After the destruction of the Second Temple in the year 70, Jews were scattered throughout the world, everywhere a minority, everywhere without rights, suffering some of the worst persecutions ever known by a people, and yet Jews survived because we never lost three things: our sense of family, our sense of community, and our faith.

And we were renewed every week especially on Shabbat, the day of rest when we give our marriages and families what they most need and are most starved of in the contemporary world, namely time. I once produced a television documentary for the BBC on the state of family life in Britain, and I took the person who was then Britain's leading expert on child care, Penelope Leach, to a Jewish primary school on a Friday morning.

There she saw the children enacting in advance what they would see that evening around the family table. There were the five-year-old mother and father blessing the five-year-old children with the five-year-old grandparents looking on. She was fascinated by this whole institution, and she asked the children what they most enjoyed about the Sabbath. One boy turned to her and said, "It's the only night of the week when daddy doesn't have to rush off." As we walked away from the school when the filming was over she turned to me and said, "Chief Rabbi, that Sabbath of yours is saving their parents' marriages."

So that is one way of telling the story, a Jewish way, beginning with the birth of sexual reproduction, then the unique demands of human parenting, then the eventual triumph of monogamy as a fundamental statement of human equality, followed by the way marriage shaped our vision of the moral and religious life as based on love and covenant and faithfulness, even to the point of thinking of truth as a conversation between lover and beloved. Marriage and the family are where faith finds its home and where the Divine Presence lives in the love between husband and wife, parent and child.

What then has changed? Here's one way of putting it. I wrote a book a few years ago about religion and science and I summarized the difference between them in two sentences. "Science takes things apart to see how they work. Religion puts things together to see what they mean." And that's a way of thinking about culture also. Does it put things together or

> **The family makes sense of the world and gives it a human face, the face of love.**

does it take things apart?

What made the traditional family remarkable, a work of high religious art, is what it brought together: sexual drive, physical desire, friendship, companionship, emotional kinship and love, the begetting of children and their protection and care, their early education and induction into an identity and a history. Seldom has any institution woven together so many different drives and desires, roles and responsibilities. It made sense of the world and gave it a human face, the face of love.

For a whole variety of reasons, some to do with medical developments like birth control, in vitro fertilization, and other genetic interventions, some to do with moral change like the idea that we are free to do whatever we like so long as it does not harm others, some to do with a transfer of responsibilities from the individual to the state, and other and more profound changes in the culture of the West, almost everything that marriage once brought together has now been split apart. Sex has been divorced from love, love from commitment, marriage from having children, and having children from responsibility for their care.

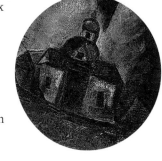

This is creating a divide within societies the like of which has not been seen since Benjamin Disraeli spoke of "two nations" a century and a half ago. Those who are privileged to grow up in stable, loving association with the two people who brought them into being will, on average, be healthier physically and emotionally. They will do better at school and at work. They will have more successful relationships, be happier, and live longer. And yes, there are many exceptions. But the injustice of it all cries out to heaven. It will go down in history as one of the tragic instances of what Friedrich Hayek called "the fatal conceit" that somehow we know better than the wisdom of the ages, and can defy the lessons of biology and history.

No one, surely, wants to go back to the narrow prejudices of the past. I think for example of the film *The Imitation Game,* which tells the story of one of the great minds of the twentieth century, Alan Turing, the Cambridge mathematician who laid the philosophical foundations of computing and artificial intelligence, and helped win the war by breaking the German naval code Enigma. After the war, Turing was arrested and tried for homosexual behavior, underwent chemically induced castration, and died at the age of forty-one by cyanide poisoning, thought by many to have committed suicide. That is a world to which we should never return.

But in our effort to create a more compassionate and inclusive society, we must not lose sight of the traditional family as the single most humanizing institution in history. The family – man, woman, and child – is not

**The family – man, woman, and child – is not one lifestyle choice among many.**

one lifestyle choice among many. It is the best means we have yet discovered for nurturing future generations and enabling children to grow in a matrix of stability and love. It is where we learn the delicate choreography of relationship and how to handle the inevitable conflicts within any human group. It is where we first take the risk of giving and receiving love. It is where one generation passes on its values to the next, ensuring the continuity of a civilization. For any society, the family is the crucible of its future, and for the sake of our children's future, we must be its defenders.

THE STORY of the first family, the first man and woman in the garden of Eden, is not generally regarded as a success. Whether or not we believe in original sin, it did not end happily. After many years of studying the text I want to suggest a different reading.

The story ends with three verses that seem to have no connection with one another. No sequence. No logic. In Genesis 3:19 God says to the man: "By the sweat of your brow you will eat your food until you return to the ground, since from it you were taken; for dust you are and to dust you will return." Then in the next verse we read: "The man named his wife Eve, because she was the mother of all life." And in the next, "The Lord God made garments of skin for Adam and his wife and clothed them."

What is the connection here? Why did God's telling the man that he was mortal lead him to give his wife a new name? And why did that act seem to change God's attitude to both of them, so that he performed an act of

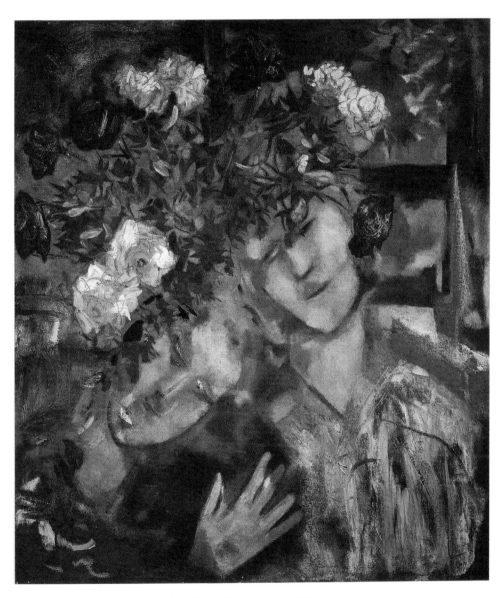

Marc Chagall, *Lovers with Flowers*, 1927

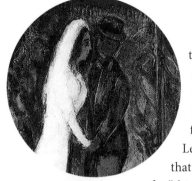

tenderness, by making them clothes, almost as if he had partially forgiven them? Let me also add that the Hebrew word for "skin" is almost indistinguishable from the Hebrew word for "light," so that Rabbi Meir, the great sage of the early second century, read the text as saying that God made for them "garments of light." What did he mean?

If we read the text carefully, we see that until now the first man had given his wife a purely generic name. He called her *ishah*, woman. Recall what he said when he first saw her: "This is now bone of my bones and flesh of my flesh; she shall be called woman for she was taken from man." For him she was a type, not a person. He gave her a noun, not a name. What is more, he defines her as a derivative of himself: something taken from man. She is not yet for him someone other, a person in her own right. She is merely a kind of reflection of himself.

As long as the man thought he was immortal, he ultimately needed no one else. But now he knew he was mortal. He would one day die and return to dust. There was only one way in which something of him would live on after his death. That would be if he had a child. But he could not have a child on his own. For that he needed his wife. She alone could give birth. She alone could mitigate his mortality. And not because she was like him but precisely because she was unlike him. At that moment she ceased to be, for him, a type, and became a person in her own right. And a person has a proper name. That is what he gave her: the name Chavah, "Eve," meaning "giver of life."

At that moment, as they were about to leave Eden and face the world as we know it, a place of darkness, Adam gave his wife the first gift of love, a personal name. And at that moment, God responded to them both in love, and made them garments to clothe their nakedness, or as Rabbi Meir put it, "garments of light."

And so it has been ever since, that when a man and woman turn to one another in a bond of faithfulness, God robes them in garments of light, and we come as close as we will ever get to God himself, bringing new life into being, turning the prose of biology into the poetry of the human spirit, redeeming the darkness of the world by the radiance of love. ⇒

> **And so it has been ever since, that when a man and woman turn to one another in a bond of faithfulness, God robes them in garments of light, and we come as close as we will ever get to God himself.**

---

*This article is adapted from Rabbi Sacks's contribution to the Plough book* Not Just Good but Beautiful: The Complementary Relationship between Man and Woman.

# Putting Marriage Second

## *How the Gospel Saves Fidelity*

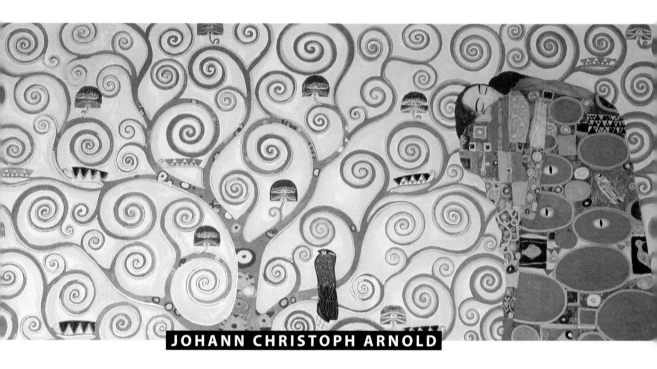

**JOHANN CHRISTOPH ARNOLD**

*Make every effort to keep the unity of the Spirit through the bond of peace.* —Ephesians 4:3

**T**RUE LOVE IS BORN of the Holy Spirit. Don't we often overlook the depth of this truth? We tend either to dismiss true love as a flimsy fairy tale or to focus so much energy on finding it that we miss it entirely. But the true love that stems from the Holy Spirit is not brought about by human effort. A married couple who experiences its blessings will notice their love increasing with each passing year, regardless of the trials they may encounter.

Decades into their marriage, they will still find joy in making each other happy.

When two people seek to have a deeper, more intimate relationship, they usually do so in terms of mutual emotions, common values, shared ideas, and a feeling of goodwill toward each other. Without despising these, we must recognize that the Holy Spirit opens up an entirely different plane of experience between husband and wife.

Certainly, marital love based on the excitement of emotion can be wonderful, but it can all too quickly become desperate and unhappy.

Gustav Klimt, *The Tree of Life*, from the *Stoclet Frieze* (1905–1911), detail

---

*Johann Christoph Arnold (1940–2017) was elder of the Bruderhof and the author of books on marriage, parenting, education, and the end of life.*

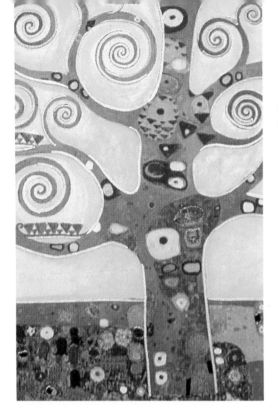

Gustav Klimt,
*The Tree of Life*,
detail

for her" (Eph. 5:25). For Christians, marriage is a reflection of the deepest unity: the unity of God and his church. In a Christian marriage, therefore, it is the unity of God's kingdom, in Christ and in the Holy Spirit, that matters most. Ultimately, it is the only sure foundation on which a marriage can be built. "Seek first God's kingdom and his righteousness, and all these things will be given to you as well" (Matt. 6:33).

Marriage should always lead two believing people closer to Jesus and his kingdom. It is not good enough for a couple to get married in a church or by a minister. To be drawn nearer to Christ, they must first be fully dedicated as individuals to the spirit of God's kingdom, and to the church community that serves it and stands under its direction. First there must be heartfelt unity of faith and spirit. Only then will there be true unity of soul and body as well. This is why (at least traditionally) so many churches have been reluctant to bless the union of a member with a spouse who does not share his or her faith in Christ (2 Cor. 6:14).

Here it should be said that the demands of a godly marriage can never be met by a human system of answers or solved by means of principles, rules, and regulations. They can be grasped only in the light of God's unity, by those who have experienced his Spirit, accepted it personally, and begun to live in accordance with it.

The very essence of God's will is unity. This is why Jesus, in his last prayer, prayed that his followers would be one, just as he and the Father were one (John 17:20–23). It was God's will for unity that brought Pentecost to the world. Through the outpouring of the Spirit, people's hearts were struck, and they repented and were baptized. The fruits of their new life were not only spiritual. The material and practical aspects of their lives, too, were affected and even revolutionized. Goods were collected

In the long run it is an unstable foundation. If we seek only the unity and love that are possible on a human level, we remain like clouds drifting and suspended. When we seek unity in the Spirit, God can ignite in us a faithful love that can endure to the end. The Spirit burns away everything that cannot endure. He purifies our love. True love does not originate from within ourselves, but is poured out over us.

In his *Confession of Faith* (1540), the Anabaptist Peter Riedemann describes God's order for marriage as encompassing three levels. First is the marriage of God to his people, of Christ to his church, and of the Spirit to our spirit (1 Cor. 6:17). Second is the community of God's people among themselves – justice and common fellowship in spirit and soul. Third is the unity between one man and one woman (Eph. 5:31), which "is visible to and understandable by all."

Paul the Apostle also draws a parallel between marriage and spiritual unity when he tells husbands to love their wives "just as Christ loved the church and gave himself up

and sold, and the proceeds were laid at the feet of the apostles. Everyone wanted to give all they had out of love. Yet no one suffered want, and everyone received what he or she needed. Nothing was held back. There were no laws or principles to govern this revolution. Not even Jesus said exactly how it should be brought about, only, "Sell your possessions and give to the poor" (Matt. 19:21). At Pentecost it simply happened: the Spirit descended and united the hearts and lives of those who believed (Acts 2:42–47).

We ourselves are not capable of bringing about the spiritual unity in which two hearts become one. That can happen only when we allow ourselves to be gripped and transformed by something greater than ourselves.

Marriage contains a mystery far deeper than the bond of husband and wife: that is, the eternal unity of Christ with his people. In a true marriage, the unity of husband and wife will reflect this deeper unity. It is not only a bond between one man and one woman, because it is sealed by the greater bond of unity with God and his people.

This bond must always come first. In my church, we affirm this unity at baptism and reaffirm it at every celebration of the Lord's Supper, and we remind ourselves of it at every wedding. How little the marriage covenant amounts to when it is only a promise or contract between two people! How different the state of the modern family would be if Christians everywhere were willing to place loyalty to Christ and his church above their marriages.

For those who have faith, Christ – the one who truly unites – always stands between the lover and the beloved. It is his Spirit that gives them unhindered access to one another. Therefore, when sin enters a marriage and clouds the truth of love, a faithful disciple will follow Jesus

in the church, not his or her wayward spouse.

Emotional love will protest this because it is prone to disregard the truth. It may even try to hinder the clear light that comes from God. It is unable and unwilling to let go of a relationship, even when it becomes false and ungenuine. But true love never follows evil: it rejoices in the truth (1 Cor. 13:6). Both marriage partners must recognize that unity of faith is more important than the emotional bond of their marriage. Each of us who claims to be a disciple must ask ourselves: "If my first allegiance is not to Jesus and the church, who is it to?" (Luke 9:57–60).

When the smaller unity of a married couple is placed under the greater unity of the church, their marriage becomes steadfast and secure on a new, deeper level because it is placed within the unity of all believers.

**True love does not originate from within ourselves, but is poured out over us.**

The conviction that love to Christ and his church must take priority over all else is also important for understanding the difference between man and woman. It has been said that the body is shaped by the soul, and this is a deep thought. The soul, the breath of God, the innermost essence of each human being, forms a different body for each. It is never a question of who is higher. Both man and woman were made in the image of God, and what can be greater than that? Yet there is a difference: Paul likens man to Christ and woman to the church (Eph. 5:22–24). Man, as head, portrays the service of Christ. Woman, as body, portrays the dedication of the church. There is a difference in calling, but there is no difference in worth.

Mary is a symbol of the church. In her we recognize the true nature of womanhood and motherhood. Woman is like the church because she receives and carries the Word within her (Luke 1:38) and brings life into the world in keeping with God's will. This is the highest thing that can be said of a human being.

It is clear, of course, that the difference between man and woman is not absolute. In

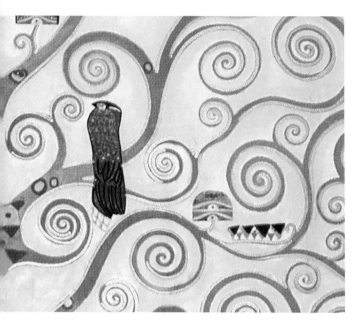

Gustav Klimt, *The Tree of Life*, detail

a true woman there is courageous manliness, and in a true man there is the submission and humility of Mary. Yet because the husband is the head, he will give the lead, even if he is a very weak person. This must not be taken as if man were an overlord and woman his servant. If a husband does not lead in love and humility – if he does not lead in the spirit of Jesus – his headship will become tyranny. The head has its place in the body, but it does not dominate.

When I marry a couple, I always ask the bridegroom if he is willing to lead his wife "in all that is good," which simply means to lead her more deeply to Jesus. In the same way, I ask

the bride if she is willing to follow her husband "in all that is good." It is simply a matter of both of them following Jesus together.

In his letter to the Ephesians, Paul points to the self-sacrificing love that lies in true leadership: to love one's spouse "just as Christ loved the church and gave himself up for her" (Eph. 5:25). This task, the task of loving, is actually the task of every man and woman, whether married or not.

When we take Paul's words to heart, we will experience the true inner unity of a relationship ruled by love – an inner speaking of the heart to God from both spouses together. Only then will God's blessing rest on our marriages. We will constantly seek our beloved one anew and continually look for ways to serve each other in love. Most wonderful of all, we will find everlasting joy. As the church father Tertullian writes:

> Who can describe the happiness of a marriage contracted in the presence of the church and sealed with its blessing? What a sweet yoke it is which here joins two believing people in one hope, one way of life, one vow of loyalty, and one service to God! They are brother and sister, both busy in the same service, with no separation of soul and body, but as two in one flesh. And where there is one flesh, there is one spirit also. Together they pray, together they kneel down: the one teaches the other, and bears with the other. They are joined together in the church of God, joined at the Lord's table, joined in anxiety, persecution, and recovery. They vie with each other in the service of their Lord. Christ sees and hears, and joyfully does he send them his peace, for where two are gathered together in his name, there is he in the midst of them. ⤳

---

*This article is adapted from Johann Christoph Arnold,* Sex, God, and Marriage *(Plough, 2014).* plough.com/sexgodandmarriage

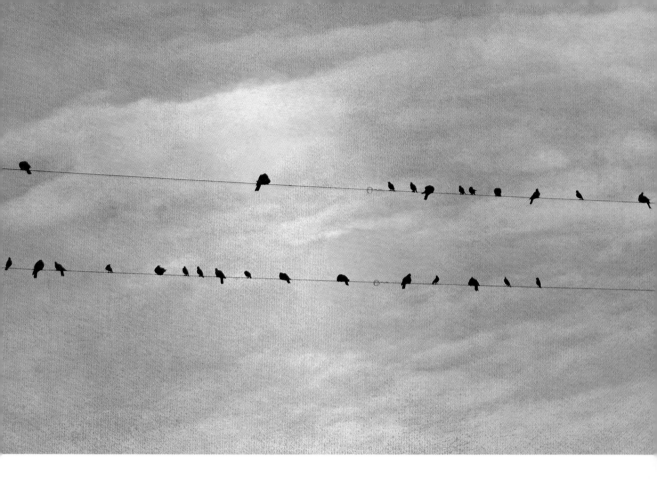

# Singles in the Pew

## *What the Unmarried Need from Church*

**GINA DALFONZO**

EASTER IS MY FAVORITE HOLIDAY. Going to church on Easter is one of my least favorite activities. This may sound as if I only love Easter for the chocolate bunnies, but that's not true. I love the religious significance – the empty tomb, the angels, the appearances of the risen Christ – all of it.

What I do not love is sitting alone in church on Easter morning. For some reason, this has happened several times now. I carefully extricate myself from nursery duty to make sure I can take part in the most joyous service of the year, only to be abruptly brought down to earth as I find that the friends I usually sit with

---

*Gina Dalfonzo is the author of* One by One: Welcoming the Singles in Your Church *(Baker, 2017) and* Dorothy and Jack: The Transforming Friendship of Dorothy L. Sayers and C. S. Lewis *(Baker, 2020), and the editor of* The Gospel in Dickens: Selections from His Works *(Plough, 2020).*

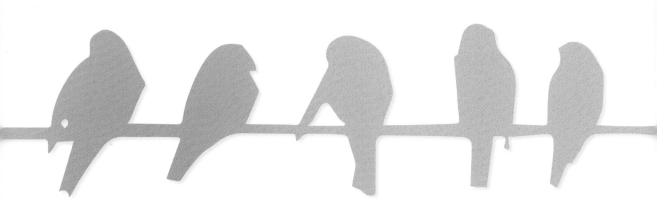

couldn't make it. Holidays do tend to cause extra work, stress, and chaos, and it's not really so surprising that many end up needing to stay home to take care of it. It is painful, however. I've even had serious thoughts of going back to the nursery in future years, to at least make myself useful.

My Easter experiences encapsulate what so many singles go through at church, not just on holidays but Sunday after Sunday. There are ways around it, of course. We can keep texting friends beforehand until we find one who will be there and can sit with us. We can come into church and ask a family to let us join them.

The hard part of it, the little ache in the heart that never quite goes away, is that we have to work constantly for the most basic companionship. Rather than facing Sunday with the knowledge that a spouse or child will be there beside us, we have to be intentional in our quest for such a presence in our lives, again and again and again.

"Intentional" is one of those terms Christian speakers and writers have overused to the point of making it a cliché. However, clichés become clichés for a reason. Intentionality is a concept we Christians really do need to apply in everyday life. As the body of Christ, it is our task to forge connections that go beyond our own family and even beyond our own community – to make brothers and sisters out of people completely unrelated to us and often very different from us. That takes all the intentionality we can muster. It does not happen naturally or quickly; it requires one deliberate act after another, for an indefinite stretch of time.

Single Christians in particular know the importance of this work, from sheer necessity. Aside from our families of origin, from whom we are often distanced, we lack the natural connections shared by the spouses and their children in the pews around us. Intentionality, for us, is a way of life.

This was brought home to me recently when I updated my will. When one has no spouse or children to whom one can leave everything, this takes a whole new level of intentionality. I spent weeks pondering the fate of my most prized possessions. This was not, I hope, out of an excess of materialism. It was because the things that mean the most to me will not become family heirlooms, as I wish they could. There is no passing them down the generations, at least not to direct descendants. There are my parents and sister, but that is more a passing up or sideways. I could have bequeathed everything to charity, but something in me could not face the thought of my things going to people who would not remember me when they wore or read or looked at them. A self-centered feeling, most likely, but I could not shake it.

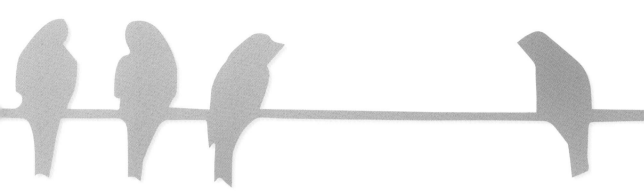

I mention this because it illustrates the extra work and creative thought that have to go into so many of the normal rituals of life for those of us without spouses or children. To create and sustain familial bonds, for us, takes an extra level of effort and an almost infinite amount of flexibility. It means learning to gracefully step back when our friends get married or have children and start to let us drift out of their day-to-day lives, while still keeping ourselves available for the times when we might be called back in. It means, in our interactions with them, orienting ourselves around their lives and interests as an acknowledgment of the many nonnegotiable demands on their time and energy, and knowing that ours, for now, must take second place.

This is our part of the bonding process. It is not easy, but it is necessary. Also, I will admit, it is good training in the selflessness that every Christian is supposed to pursue.

The part of our married friends is to find a way to continue making space for us in their hectic lives, and that is not easy either. "She who is married cares about the things of the world – how she may please her husband," as Paul reminds us. And how she may please her children, he might have added. Spouses and parents are constantly practicing their own very necessary forms of selflessness, often with little to spare outside the bounds of their family.

On both sides – singles and married couples – we're doing the difficult task of creating a family relationship based not just on the natural needs, demands, and connections of actual family, but on the call of Christ to be mutually helpful and mutually dependent members of his body.

New Testament scholars have noted how frequently Paul portrays the relationship between Christians as one between brothers and sisters. At a time when life expectancy was short and many children lost their parents early, siblingship was deeply important. In that world, siblings were expected to care for each other, advocate for each other, respect each other, and provide for each other.

This is the kind of relationship Paul had in mind when he referred to men in the church as brothers and women as sisters. It was no light or casual reference; instead, it was one of the strongest he could have used. This tightest of bonds, he was saying, is the kind of bond that should hold Christians together. This is the relationship to which Christ calls us.

I'm sure Jesus knew this task would not be easy when he gave it to us, but he gave it

**We must make brothers and sisters out of people completely unrelated to us and often very different from us.**

anyway. He gave it because he wanted to give the world a picture of what true community looks like, to show that in him our natural bonds are transcended and new bonds are created, bonds that are capable of including and holding the lonely, the needy, the outsiders. In him there is a family that is more than family.

But to get there, to show this picture to the world, we have to do the work.

**We need the spiritual siblings that God made provision for when he established his church.**

This is where intentionality comes in. To keep others in our lives, to keep doing the hard work of friendship – or more, of creating the family of God – it is necessary to keep pushing past the dozens of barriers life keeps throwing in our way. It is necessary to make the decision every day to reach out, to send the text or make the phone call, to extend the invitation to lunch, to ask if there are any needs, to pray, to consider, to remember, to care.

Christians who are single and childless, in my experience, are more inclined to do this work simply because we are so much more dependent on the church to be our family. Except for cases when our family of origin is nearby and available, we cannot fall back on the natural family bonds that sustain others. We must be forever busy building, strengthening, reinforcing the bonds with those outside our family – and most importantly, with fellow members of the church. We may be tempted to form our strongest friendships at work, forgetting how easily those bonds can break when other employees leave the company or when we leave ourselves, confusing the professional with the personal in ways that may not always be healthy. We need the spiritual siblings that God made provision for when he established

his church. But the church – in particular, the married majority of the church – has not always stepped up for us.

"Being a single woman (especially without children) puts you out of sync with your peers in a way that's particularly hard on friendship," says my friend Ruth Buchanan, author of *The Proper Care and Feeding of Singles*. "All friendships require sacrifice, attention, and intentionality. . . . But this dynamic persists." Her plea to married people: "Invite singles into your family's rhythms. In God's plan, we all need one another."

This is truer than many married people realize. The number of married people who have told me that they feel lonely even within their marriages demonstrates that the married need friends too. They need people around them who can listen to their struggles and offer an objective point of view, who can be the cool "aunt" or "uncle" in their children's lives, who can talk with them about things outside the family and help them take a broader perspective. They also need to learn to prepare themselves for the day when the family unit is no longer the family unit it was – when the children leave the nest, when only one spouse is left, or even when one spouse decides to stop coming to church, leaving the other to sit alone in a pew week after week. They need friends who know such experiences well and can sympathize and help. For all these reasons, the married need the single.

The good thing is that the single already know how to be there for them. Through the lessons we've learned from this difficult and intentional work, we can lead the way in this area. It only requires a willingness on the part of others to acknowledge our presence and our value, to make space for us in their lives – and to keep a seat for us in the pew. ➤

# New Prince, New Pompe

## ROBERT SOUTHWELL

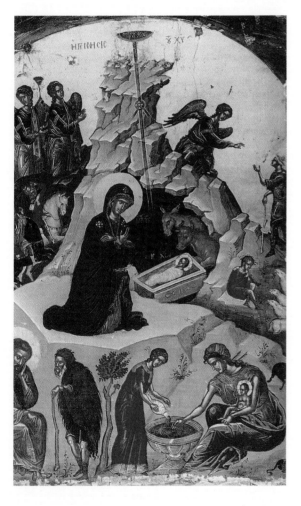

Behould a sely tender Babe,
In freesing winter nighte,
In homely manger trembling lies;
Alas, a pitious sighte!

The inns are full, no man will yelde
This little pilgrime bedd;
But forc'd He is with sely beastes
In cribb to shroude His headd.

This stable is a Prince's courte,
The cribb His chaire of State;
The beastes are parcell of His pompe,
The wodden dish His plate.

The persons in that poore attire
His royall liveries weare;
The Prince Himself is come from heaven,
This pompe is prisèd there.

With joy approch, O Christian wighte!
Do homage to thy Kinge;
And highly prise His humble pompe
Which He from heaven doth bringe.

Icon of the Nativity of Christ by Theophanes the Cretan, 1546

Source: Alexander Balloch Grossart, ed., *The Complete Poems of Robert Southwell* (England: private circulation, 1872), 107.

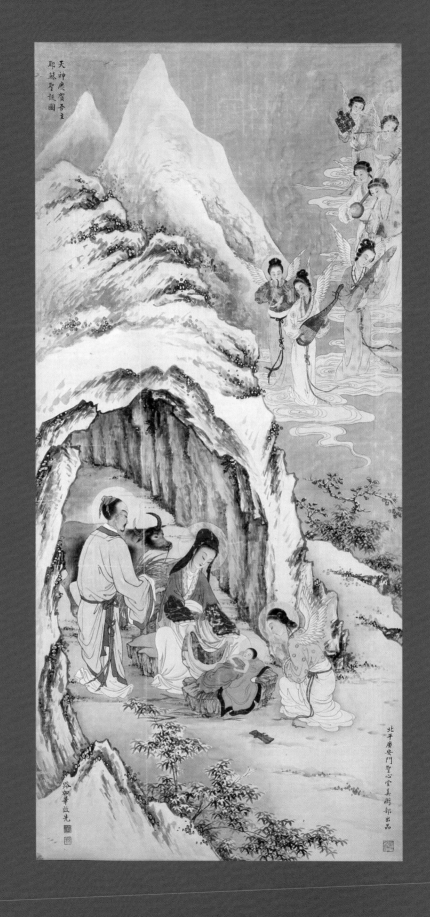

# God in a Cave

## A Reading on the Holy Family

G. K. CHESTERTON

**T**HE OLD TRINITY was of father and mother and child and is called the human family. The new is of child and mother and father and has the name of the Holy Family. It is in no way altered except in being entirely reversed; just as the world which is transformed was not in the least different, except in being turned upside down.

This sketch of the human story began in a cave; the cave which popular science associates with the caveman and in which practical discovery has really found archaic drawings of animals. The second half of human history, which was like a new creation of the world, also begins in a cave. There is even a shadow of such a fancy in the fact that animals were again present; for it was a cave used as a stable by the mountaineers of the uplands about Bethlehem; who still drive their cattle into such holes and caverns at night. It was here that a homeless couple had crept underground with the cattle when the doors of the crowded caravanserai had been shut in their faces; and it was here beneath the very feet of the passers-by, in a cellar under the very floor of the world, that Jesus Christ was born. But in that second creation there was indeed something symbolical in the roots of the primeval rock or the horns of the prehistoric

*Opposite:*
Hua Xiaoxian,
*The Nativity,*
1948

---

G. K. Chesterton (1874–1936) was an English writer, philosopher, lay theologian, and literary and art critic. Abridged excerpt from *The Everlasting Man* (Hodder & Stoughton, 1925), 201–207.

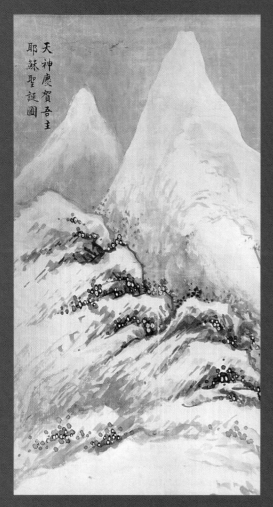

天神慶賀吾主
耶穌聖誕圖

as remote from each other; the idea of a baby and the idea of unknown strength that sustains the stars. His instincts and imagination can still connect them, when his reason can no longer see the need of the connection; for him there will always be some savor of religion about the mere picture of a mother and a baby; some hint of mercy and softening about the mere mention of the dreadful name of God. . . . There is really a difference between the man who knows it and the man who does not.

It might be suggested, in a somewhat violent image, that nothing had happened in that fold or crack in the great grey hills except that the whole universe had been turned inside out. I mean that all the eyes of wonder and worship which had been turned outwards to the largest thing were now turned inward to the smallest.

Whether as a myth or a mystery, Christ was obviously conceived as born in a hole in the rocks primarily because it marked the position of one outcast and homeless. Nevertheless it is true, as I have said, that the cave has not been so commonly or so clearly used as a symbol as the other realities that surrounded the first Christmas.

And the reason for this also refers to the very nature of that new world. It was in a sense the difficulty of a new dimension. Christ was not only born on the level of the world, but even lower than the world. The first act of the divine drama was enacted, not only on no stage set up above the sight-seer, but on a dark and curtained stage sunken out of sight; and that is an idea very difficult to express in most modes of artistic expression.

But in the riddle of Bethlehem it was heaven that was under the earth. There is in that alone the touch of a revolution, as of the world turned upside down. ⤳

herd. God also was a caveman, and had also traced strange shapes of creatures, curiously colored, upon the wall of the world; but the pictures that he made had come to life.

A mass of legend and literature, which increases and will never end, has repeated and rung the changes on that single paradox; that the hands that had made the sun and stars were too small to reach the huge heads of the cattle.

**A**NY AGNOSTIC OR ATHEIST whose childhood has known a real Christmas has ever afterwards, whether he likes it or not, an association in his mind between two ideas that most of mankind must regard

# Editors' Picks

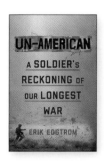

### Un-American
A Soldier's Reckoning of Our Longest War

*Erik Edstrom*
*(Bloomsbury)*

Every reckoning of debt requires an accounting. Of course, not all debts are simply economic; some require us to use our moral imaginations to measure what we owe. What do we owe someone to whom we've lied? What do we owe the victim of a crime? Or, to take a slightly more complicated example which most Americans ignore, what are the true costs of America's "forever war" in the Middle East?

West Point alumnus and former Army officer Erik Edstrom wrestles with that question in this incisive memoir. He offers three ways one can begin to come to grips with the reality of US military presence in the Middle East: through an honest assessment of the war's price tag in material terms and in opportunities lost by diverting resources to its mission, by imagining one's own death in the war, and by imagining what it would be like to be subjected to a foreign occupying force here at home.

Don't think that *Un-American* is a straightforward polemic. Edstrom pulls us into his life story, taking us along as he comes of age in blue-collar Massachusetts, succumbs to a pervasive jingoism as a high school student after 9/11, and is transformed into an unquestioning soldier at West Point. "One day...I crossed a line. I was now capable of hunting people. Not only that, I was looking forward

to it." Coming face to face with the actual evils of war – the charred bodies, the pointless missions, the skewed moral reasoning, and the pompous propaganda – gradually awakens Edstrom from the brainwashing of American militarism. "I was very lucky," he writes, "I compromised my morals and had the formative years of my life amputated by serving in an unnecessary war," yet survived to tell the tale.

So how do we reckon our war debt? The price in material terms and lost opportunities should be obvious. "America," Edstrom writes, "has lost a chance to adequately deal with far larger threats, starting with the climate crises and followed by other important issues, including technological surveillance and data rights, AI and vocational retraining, infrastructure, education, health care, and wealth equality." But even more powerfully, Edstrom asks us to put ourselves in the shoes of our so-called enemies, with a foreign force invading our own towns: "They...throw water bottles filled with urine at children. They disrespect your religion. They kill anyone in your community who actively fights back in self-defense." They torture and raze and still have the audacity to tell you that they're "only here to help, to free the oppressed."

*Un-American* trenchantly questions the lack of moral vision in tabulating the cost of America's longest war. It's every bit as critical as anything by esteemed academics, while written in accessible language and hewing closer to the bone of lived experience. We owe it to ourselves to read it.

*—Scott Beauchamp, author,*
*Did You Kill Anyone?*

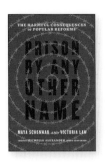

## Prison by Any Other Name
The Harmful Consequences of Popular Reforms

*Maya Schenwar and Victoria Law*
*(The New Press)*

Journalists Schenwar and Law deliver a thorough deconstruction of a system they are convinced should not be reformed but abolished and replaced with an entirely reimagined approach to crime and justice. Though what they propose may seem extreme to some, even skeptics will benefit from reconsidering why our society keeps 2.3 million people locked up and many more under supervision and surveillance.

Law and Schenwar give a deep analysis of the harm inflicted through many so-called criminal justice reform efforts, which might reduce the number of people behind literal bars while in fact expanding the carceral net throughout our lives – into our homes, our communities, and our work until we find ourselves living in a prison nation.

The question driving Law and Schenwar's analysis is "What is a prison?" They find that the state's appetite for controlling citizens' lives, enhanced by technological solutions and combined with a punitive approach to crime and poverty, already infects society well beyond the prison system. Specifically, the book explores probation, electronic monitoring, departments of child services, community policing, and the carceral nature of schools and drug treatment programs to reveal a landscape that under the guise of reform has grown the prison nation exponentially. The authors analyze the past several decades, during which a growing awareness of mass incarceration began to shift cultural awareness and the broader conversation around incarceration away from tough-on-crime to "smart-on-crime" rhetoric through the strange bedfellow alliances of the Koch brothers, the NAACP, and the Center for American Progress, to name just a few.

Commendably, the authors actually lay out a fairly detailed proposal for abolition and all it would encompass, offering concrete suggestions, not ephemeral dreams. This is a book to be taken seriously by everyone who cares about what transformative justice might look like.

*—Jeannie Alexander, founder, No Exceptions Prison Collective*

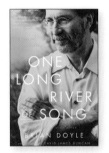

## One Long River of Song
Notes on Wonder for the Spiritual and Nonspiritual Alike

*Brian Doyle*
*(Little, Brown)*

If you're not familiar with Oregon novelist and essayist Brian Doyle, think James Joyce, but with earnest faith. Joyce was haunted by his Catholicism, and it permeates his work. Doyle was also haunted by his faith, but in his writing that haunting blooms into joy, wonder, and some of the most agile, inspiring sentences in recent memory.

These collected essays are a posthumous gift to the world – Doyle died in 2017 of a brain tumor – and are as much performances of syntax as they are spiritual pilgrimages. Start at the perfectly placed first piece, "Joyas Voladoras," a meditation on our mortal, weak hearts: "So much held in a heart in a lifetime." In "Two Hearts," he is angry at the God who caused one of his twin sons to be born with a heart condition – but knows "that this same

God made my magic boys, shaped their apple faces and coyote eyes, put joy in the eager suck of their mouths."

Doyle writes of flora and fauna, of childhood and basketball and pants and anesthesiologists and love – of all things we will miss, or already miss. His essays are apologias in both senses of the word – playful treatises that demonstrate the blessings of belief, and self-effacing jaunts through his own faults. Conversational and cathartic, Doyle has managed to give words to that epiphanic rush we feel when we catch a glimpse of the divine.

—*Nick Ripatrazone, culture editor,*
*Image Journal*

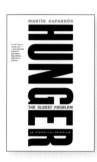

### Hunger
### The Oldest Problem

*Martín Caparrós*
*Translated from the Spanish*
*by Katherine Silver*
*(Melville House)*

Right at this moment, eight hundred million people suffer from hunger. Twenty-five thousand die of hunger every day while one third of food produced worldwide goes to waste. In this meticulously researched book, Martín Caparrós asks why, and what we can do about it.

Caparrós travels to Niger, India, Bangladesh, the United States, Argentina, South Sudan, and Madagascar to talk with the poorest people on earth. They tell him about their daily lives: how they find food, what they eat, and why they struggle to get enough. He finds that those who suffer chronic malnutrition often do not realize it. Just-weaned children die in all these regions because they cannot make it on the nutrition-poor diet of their parents. Repeatedly parents tell Caparrós that they cannot understand why their children died; they fed them every day.

A hungry person, Caparrós notes, is someone you can exploit. Thus there are those who benefit from hunger, from speculators who steal land from traditional farmers to corporations such as Monsanto that entice farmers to go into debt to buy genetically modified seed rather than using seed they've saved themselves. Driven to desperation, farmers in India drink the very pesticide that buried them in debt. Meanwhile, powerful global institutions such as the IMF and World Bank regularly make decisions that redirect money away from efforts to feed the poor.

Caparrós tells us that the 375 pounds of corn needed to create enough ethanol to fill one tank of gas would feed a child in Zambia or Mexico or Bangladesh for an entire year. In another section he notes that in the United States, three dollars buys three hundred calories of fruit and vegetables or 4,500 calories of french fries, cookies, and soda, making the overweight and the malnourished victims of the same hunger industry.

Woven throughout the book is a detailed history of world response to hunger. Westerners are easily misled by statistics that are adjusted to make it look as if the problem were improving. "Numbers are the alibi for pathetic relativism," Caparrós states – as long as we feel the situation is being addressed, we don't develop the outrage needed to galvanize a response. We are, he writes, at a moment in history "when the previous paradigm has broken down, and another one has yet to appear." He views that as reason for hope: with vision, leadership, and real struggles, the world's oldest problem can be addressed.

—*Suzanne Quinta, Fox Hill Bruderhof*

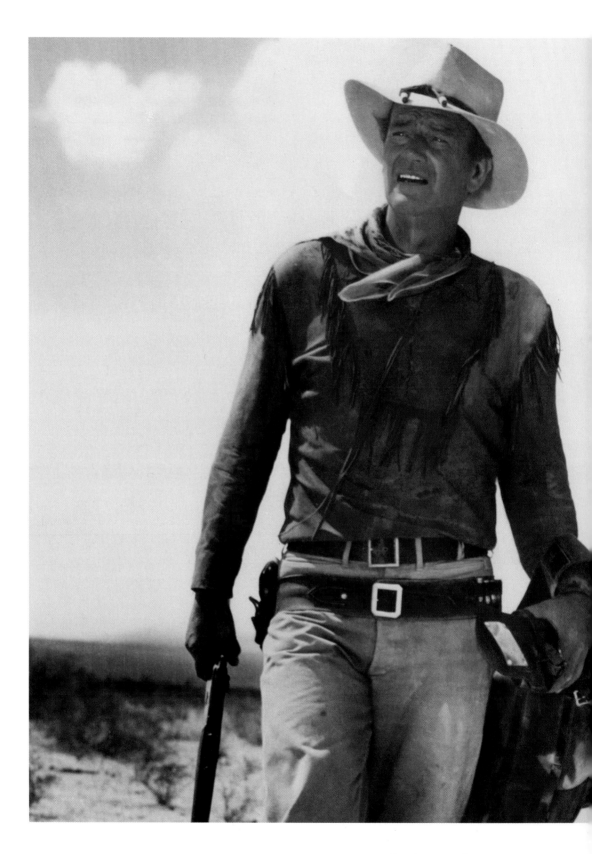

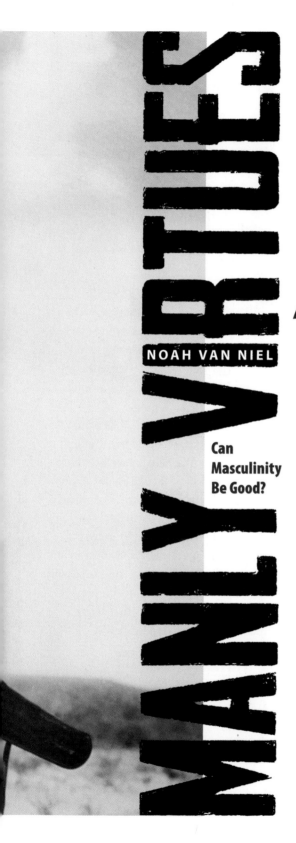

# MANLY VIRTUES

**NOAH VAN NIEL**

**Can Masculinity Be Good?**

"**S**ING ABOUT THAT, BITCH!" he spat, pushing my helmet into the turf. I made sure I'd cleared the first-down marker, tossed the ball to the referee, and jogged back toward the huddle, chuckling. Their linebacker had done his homework – news had recently broken that Harvard's starting fullback was also an aspiring opera singer, and my resulting fifteen minutes of fame were easily discoverable by our opponents.

But as press coverage spread, it became clear that when people asked, "How can you do both those things?" they didn't mean "How do you find the time?" or "How did you develop such diverse interests?" They wanted to know how I, a man, could do two seemingly antithetical things. Football players are tough and aggressive, manly; opera singers soft and effeminate. You can't be both.

This is, of course, untrue. A number of football players have turned to careers in opera, many much more accomplished than I ever was. But the question wasn't really about football or opera. It was about what it means to be a man. Over the years this sort of debate about masculinity has had many iterations, but recently it has become a full-blown crisis of identity.

John Wayne
in the film
*Hondo,* 1953

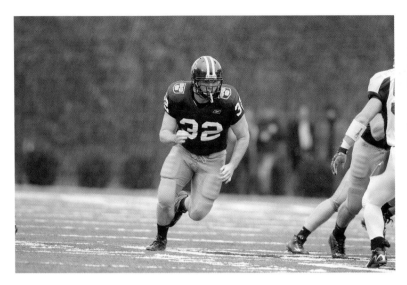
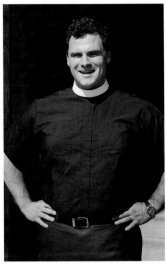

The author as starting fullback for Harvard *(left)* and Episcopal priest *(right)*

In 2019, the American Psychological Association (APA) designated "traditional" masculinity as harmful. The APA described "a particular constellation of standards that have held sway over large segments of the population, including anti-femininity, achievement, eschewal of the appearance of weakness, and adventure, risk, and violence" that have led to increased rates of suicide, substance abuse, violent behavior, unwillingness to seek medical or psychological help, and premature death for men. "Traditional" masculinity – or "toxic masculinity," in the now-common phrase – was killing us.

In establishing these guidelines, the APA was coming out strongly on one side of a contentious debate. That men were in crisis was not news. In her 2010 *Atlantic* cover story "The End of Men," Hanna Rosin explored ways men were falling behind women in education and career achievement. Others have since written articles and books exploring cultural and biological factors that might explain men's dysfunction – for example, their brain development and learning styles, or their testosterone

levels and natural aggressive tendencies. Perhaps it has to do with overbearing mothers and absent fathers, or with Hollywood movies and violent video games. Maybe it's ease of access to online pornography, or the militant feminism that makes men feel like criminals before they do anything wrong.

This debate occurred in the midst of new conversations around gender identity and sexual orientation that added nuance to those topics but also left some men confused about how they fit into this new spectrum of gender fluidity. Meanwhile, through the #MeToo movement, women courageously exposed patterns of sexual harassment and abuse by men in many corners of society. The movement was long overdue, but swift in its coming, leaving many men unsure how to navigate a rapidly shifting cultural landscape.

## JOHN WAYNE MASCULINITY

But was "traditional" masculinity as diagnosed by the APA really to blame? Or was it actually the overthrow of masculinity that robbed men of their self-confidence and

---

*Noah Van Niel is an Episcopal priest currently serving at The Chapel of the Cross in Chapel Hill, North Carolina, where he lives with his wife and two children. His sermons, writing, and other work can be found at* The Vicar's View. *thevicarsview.com*

left them confused about what it meant to be a man? In recent years, many have reverted to the "traditional" model as an ideal to be recovered, not a distortion to be rejected. It is perhaps emblematic of our divided times that John Wayne – the steel-jawed tough guy of mid-century war movies and westerns – has reentered the conversation as an ideological Rorschach test. For some he represents everything right and good about how to be male. For others he is everything that is wrong, toxic, and detrimental.

Defenders of John Wayne masculinity have been having something of a moment. The election of Donald Trump seemed to legitimize the resurgence of the tough-guy machismo so familiar from US history since its inception. In 2016, as #MeToo hit the headlines and women's marches the streets, many men retreated online to nurse their wounds and try to sort out a way forward. Over the past four years, the internet has made major celebrities of a new generation of psychospiritual gurus trying to reiterate and recover traditional masculinity. No one exemplifies this trend more than Jordan Peterson, a Canadian polymath who promises men a treasure map to meaning.

What makes Peterson alluring to many men? From outside his fan club looking in, what's striking is that he does more than just reject identity politics and political correctness: he promises to bring order to the chaos men find themselves in. Confusion seeks out clarity; crisis begs for commandments. So Peterson came up with clear steps for people to follow; his book *12 Rules for Life: An Antidote to Chaos* has sold over three million copies. You don't need to endorse all of Peterson's prescriptions, grounded as they are in his gender-essentialist views and in Jungian psychology, to recognize the power of what he offers to so many confused young men.

Peterson's rise in popularity helped expose the reality that it's far easier to deconstruct John Wayne–style manliness than it is to replace it. Those who classify "traditional" masculinity as "toxic" seem reluctant to put forth a constructive alternative, and not without reason. In their view, articulating any definition of *non*-toxic masculinity would be inherently reductive: to speak to men *as men* and not as individuals, they would say, is unavoidably to shore up a gender binary that should be dismantled.

Yet in the absence of positive alternative visions of masculinity, the vacuum has been filled by those who speak with force and clarity – for better or (more often) for worse. There is a growing audience not just for people like Peterson, but also for more troubling voices like that of Gavin McInnes, whose Proud Boys organization has traveled the slippery road from encouraging male empowerment to backing white male supremacy.

**Christianity has joined – and sometimes led – the movement back toward John Wayne–style masculinity.**

## MEN IN CHURCH

One hard-to-ignore development of recent decades is how Christianity has joined – and sometimes led – the movement toward an impoverished and brittle understanding of masculinity. One place this can be found is in the "men's ministries" or the "men's movement" in American Christianity, specifically in its Evangelical arm. More generally, Evangelicals' theological understanding of patriarchal authority, complementary gender roles, and heterosexuality allows them to speak strongly on issues of gender in a way that gives them outsize influence. And indeed, for over a century, Evangelicals have been fighting to make their men spiritual warriors in the traditional, patriarchal mode of militant masculinity.

This is the argument the historian Kristin Kobes Du Mez makes in her new book *Jesus and John Wayne.* According to Du Mez, one should understand the masculinity promoted by Evangelical Christianity as motivated culturally just as much as it is theologically and biblically. Evangelicals concluded early on that the postmodern world, with its shift from the industrial to the intellectual economy, was stripping men of their God-given roles as providers and protectors. But in seeking to counteract this, Evangelical Christianity ended up promoting an ideal of the Christian man that had much more in common with the macho ideals of popular culture than it had with Jesus Christ. Influential Evangelical leaders such as James Dobson, Pat Robertson, and Jerry Falwell unabashedly glorified culturally defined masculine attributes, seeking to make Christian men rugged, aggressive GI Joes for Jesus. Through TV, radio, books, pamphlets, and conferences, this view of masculinity spread. To be sure, there were groups that offered a different vision – Promisekeepers, which had its heyday in the 1990s, perhaps most notably – but it appears they were effectively drowned out.

Whether or not one agrees with Du Mez's wider argument, she is right to point out that the Jesus of the Gospels proves an inconvenient stumbling block to those promoting ideals of patriarchal, aggressive, militant, dominant masculinity. So those drawn to the idea of Christ-as-badass are forced to look elsewhere. They tend to emphasize not Jesus the man but the cosmic Christ, the eternal judge to whom all powers submit and obey: a figure more in the mold of John's Revelation than his Gospel. And, of course, they are keen to pick up on the warrior heroes of the Old Testament.

Accordingly, these Christians rail against the "sissified Sunday School Jesus" of mainline Protestantism – what megachurch pastor Mark Driscoll called the "Richard Simmons, hippie, queer Christ." For Driscoll, Jesus was "an Ultimate Fighter warrior king with a tattoo down his leg who rides into battle against Satan, sin, and death on a trusty horse." According to Du Mez, it's no coincidence that in 2016, 81 percent of white Evangelicals voted for Donald Trump, who claims to embody many aspects of this militant masculinity, nor that Trump was endorsed by John Wayne's daughter.

To the extent that Du Mez is right, Christian masculinity has been defined more by culture than by scripture – and so it has little to offer men beyond the toxicities of the "traditional" model.

## BEHOLD THE MAN

But Christianity does have more to offer. It has at its core the person of Jesus Christ, God made *man.* Turning away from his personhood leaves Christian men without a compelling alternative; turning toward it offers growth through a masculinity emphasizing compassion, humility, and purpose.

*Compassion:* Compassion is Jesus' driving force. Repeatedly the Gospels tell us that he is motivated by compassion: for the sick, the suffering, and the sinful. He never refuses someone who comes to him in need – Jew, Samaritan, or Roman; man, woman, or child.

> **The Jesus of the Gospels proves an inconvenient stumbling block to those promoting ideals of patriarchal, aggressive, militant, dominant masculinity.**

Emulating Christlike compassion requires care for others: friends, strangers, enemies. It requires showing mercy and granting forgiveness; to Jesus no one is beyond redemption. Compassion leads men to be healers and helpers rather than dominators or destroyers.

It also requires cultivating an emotional openness that allows one to feel the sorrow and pain of others. Emotional detachment, stoicism, the repression of feelings – some of those "traditional" male qualities the APA warned against – are the antithesis of compassion. Jesus wept at the death of his friend Lazarus. He admitted when he was afraid: "I am deeply grieved, even unto death," he tells his friends (Matt. 26:38). By learning from Jesus' emotional intelligence and using it to connect deeply with others, a Jesus-based masculinity encourages availability in personal and professional relationships and openness to the richness at the heart of Christian life.

*Humility:* Humility was another cornerstone of Jesus' life. "All who exalt themselves will be humbled and those who humble themselves will be exalted" (Luke 14:11). The value he accorded humility increased his anger at the scribes and Pharisees he thought were greedy and self-indulgent, seeking places of honor at the table and making public shows of their piety. Instead, he says, "the greatest among you will be your servant" (Matt. 23:11). That is what he models for his disciples by washing their feet the night before his death, and it is how he understands his mission: "The Son of Man came not to be served, but to serve, and to give his life a ransom for many" (Matt. 20:28).

Jesus doesn't use his power to show off or control others; he rejects Satan's offer of the splendors of the world. His power is for the powerless, made great by being given away. To the poor, the oppressed, and the persecuted he proclaims, "Yours is the kingdom of heaven."

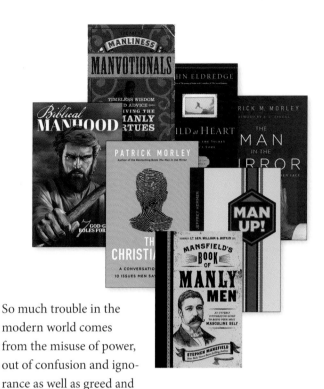

So much trouble in the modern world comes from the misuse of power, out of confusion and ignorance as well as greed and lust. Jesus offers a clear way out: if we do as he does, we will renounce the drive for supremacy and dominance, stop glorifying our own strength and authority, and pursue humility and service, lifting up others, not ourselves.

*Purpose:* One shouldn't make the mistake of thinking humility means passivity and weakness. Jesus worked hard, traveling the countryside so people could hear and follow him: "My mother and my brothers are those who hear the word of God and do it" (Luke 8:21). He wants people to bear good fruit; to multiply the gifts they have been given, not bury them in the ground. He wasn't afraid to offer a harsh word or to point out hypocrisy and injustice. But he was also patient. He invited people to follow him; he didn't force them. He was willing to listen to those he disagreed with and to engage in debate with them. He refused to fight them physically because he knew that "all who take the sword will perish by the sword" (Matt. 26:52). To call such a man weak is to mistake peacefulness for passivity, sacrifice for surrender. There is nothing weak about the cross.

The last three decades have brought a spate of books on Christian manhood.

Some men have responded to today's confusion with loss of purpose or malaise – they've been called the "omega" males, the "failsons." They give up on school, give up on jobs, fall into slothful routines, and don't seem to care much about anything or anyone. Jesus offers men a purpose that calls them out of themselves to serve others – without letting that purpose become another instrument for control.

## A HIGHER CHALLENGE

Compassion, humility, and purpose are only a few of the qualities Jesus asks us to embrace. His honesty and integrity would discourage the lying, cheating, and stealing that infect many men's hearts and poison their relationships. His pacifism would be a powerful response to the glorification of violence and aggression. His faithfulness to God might help men who are drifting from organized religion. His lack of attachment to worldly goods could help them resist connecting their self-worth to paychecks or possessions. And his commitment to combating injustice could inspire more men to use their privilege to fight for those with less.

> **The world does not reward men for being like Jesus – it certainly didn't reward Jesus for being like Jesus.**

Looking closely at the man Jesus shows us how far we have strayed. But it also makes clear his offer of a new way – in fact a very old way – of conceiving what a man should be.

Following Jesus will always be harder than following a Jordan Peterson. He calls men not only to swim against the cultural tide but to overcome what they have been told are irresistible drives for domination and sex. The world does not reward men for being like Jesus – it certainly didn't reward Jesus for being like Jesus. You won't get paid much, you won't get famous, you won't get the riches of this life by walking the way of Christ.

But you will become free. Jesus, God made man, shows us a way to transcend our baser selves and find a fuller, happier, healthier life. For Christian men who are desperate for guidance to chart a way in the modern world, the key is rooting their masculinity where the lives of all Christians should be based: in the timeless truth of Jesus Christ.

My football and singing days are long over. The path of my life has led to new, even more fulfilling roles as husband, father, and priest. They may not be as newsworthy, but they repeatedly call me to consider the kind of man I want to be, and the kind of men I want to encourage others to be. I have two sons. It will be a challenge to teach them how to be men in this world, particularly men of faith. I want to tell them how to be while still giving them enough space to figure out who they are. How do I allow them to love knocking over piled-up blocks but make clear that real violence and destruction are things they should avoid? How do I keep alive the fun of wrestling and competing and yet make sure domination and winning don't become too large a focus? How do I respect their emotions but encourage them to stop crying when someone takes a toy?

And this is all happening before they are affected by the wider culture, long before their testosterone kicks in. I want them to love being boys and men; I want them to be loving boys and men. I want them to thrive in this world and contribute to it. But most of that lies beyond my control. So instead of fretting about what kind of men they turn out to be, perhaps the best thing I can do for them is to introduce them to Jesus Christ and let them hear for themselves his ageless call, "Follow me." ⤜

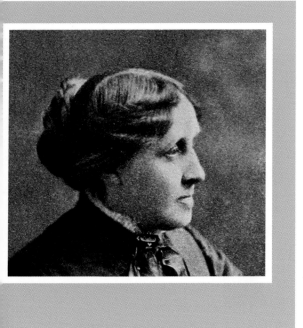

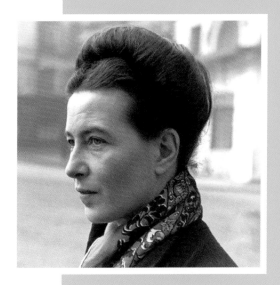

# Little Women, Rebel Angels

## *Louisa May Alcott and Simone de Beauvoir*

**MARY TOWNSEND**

SIMONE DE BEAUVOIR was not born an atheist; rather, she became one. In an inversion of Pascal's Wager, the idea of any bargain with God seemed to her to be petty and beside the point. In her 1958 autobiography, *Memoirs of a Dutiful Daughter*, she writes: "I could not admit any kind of compromise argument with heaven. However little you withheld from him, it would be too much if God existed; and however little you gave him, it would be too much again if he did not exist." The logic of all or nothing was the only logic that satisfied.

Born in 1908, Beauvoir grew up in the thick emotive haze of leftover nineteenth-century French Catholicism, carried into pre-war France. She was educated in the same sort of immersive religiosity that provided plenty of opportunities for spiritual heroism from very young girls in particular, the same sort of upbringing that produced Saint Thérèse of Lisieux, the Little Flower, who aspired to

---

*Mary Townsend is an assistant professor at St. John's University, Department of Philosophy. She is the author of* The Woman Question in Plato's Republic *(Lexington, 2017).*

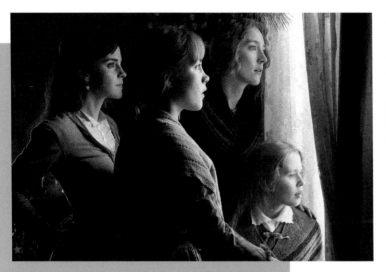

Alcott's wildly popular 1868 novel, *Little Women*. Beauvoir couldn't quite escape the nineteenth century after all.

LIKE SO MANY READERS, the young Simone was passionately invested in the persona of Jo as a writer, taking up the genre of the short story to imitate her. Inevitably, she also had extremely strong opinions on the Laurie question, the wealthy neighbor who proposes to one and then another of the March sisters. Opening the second volume *Good Wives* by accident, she came upon Laurie and Amy's engagement (without the help of Jo's refusal for context), and her response was immediate and absolute: "I hated Louisa M. Alcott for it." But the similarities between the Marches' style of family life (fictionalized from Alcott's own experience) and her own gave her pleasure: "they were taught, as I was, that a cultivated mind and moral righteousness was better than money." This was something to hold on to, the more so because like the Marches, and like Alcott herself, Beauvoir's family dealt with straitened means, the memory of better times, and the all-too-visible wealth and comfort of neighbors and relations. The reward of their virtue was to be found in the causes they took up: for Alcott, abolitionism and suffrage, and for Beauvoir, existentialism, Marxism, and her own variety of existentialist Marxist feminism. The necessity for strict social circumspection in the behavior of daughters was lost on Simone, Louisa, and Jo alike.

This funny crisscross between Alcott and Beauvoir's lives continues to tease at my sense

Stills from the 2019 film adaptation of *Little Women* by Greta Gerwig

sainthood from her very early youth and in her death in 1897. Beauvoir, who for several years aspired to be a nun, writes of the exquisite transports of confessional tears, imagining herself swooning in the arms of angels; she prided herself on inventing mortifications in her very few moments alone. But unlike Thérèse, Beauvoir found no lasting comfort within or even distantly alongside Christianity.

It was not by cutting herself off from transports of emotion or by abandoning the metaphysical all-or-nothing that she eventually found an image of adulthood she could live with; nor could the attractions of philosophy, which she first came across through the Thomism of her girls' school, or the Catholic social justice group she volunteered for, do the trick. It was rather literature, as a kind of Art, and herself as Author, that managed to hold the strongest and most sustainable appeal as vocation. If you can believe it, the first non-saintly individual Beauvoir found really attractive was the fictional American Protestant, Jo March, one of the heroines of Louisa May

of the significant, with the added coincidence of the Greta Gerwig film and a new biography of Beauvoir from Kate Kirkpatrick, both coming out in the last year. The film is lovely, although I'm somewhat distant from it as a fan; I, too, read *Little Women* with pleasure in my youth, but it never seemed the reflection or the idealization of my childhood. In fact, it was only when I read Beauvoir's *Memoirs of a Dutiful Daughter* that I had a reading experience analogous to what many report about Alcott, where the author's descriptions seem to correspond to or call forth some memory of my own. I grew up in the former French colony of Louisiana, in the post-Vatican II Roman church; like Beauvoir, I had one younger sister, one devout parent and one more skeptical, a large extended family to visit, a white dress at first communion, and the confessional ready to absolve even the smallest of the week's sins. Alcott's landscape, by contrast, was foreign to me. That the Marches pay such close attention to regretting faults in their behavior, that they give up wine (give up wine *for life, not even at a wedding*), that they worry over whether they've allowed their passions too much sway – all of these are fundamentally un-French attitudes taken by no adult I knew well. To me, the Protestant world of *Little Women* read as fantasy.

To me, the Protestant world of *Little Women* read as fantasy.

SIMONE ALSO FINDS the Marches' Protestantism somewhat puzzling, the one wrinkle in their otherwise close correspondence. She read *Little Women* in English; the French translation converts Mr. March into a doctor, the better not to scandalize its readers with married clergy. The Marches had their *Pilgrim's Progress*, but Beauvoir's mother gave her Thomas à Kempis's *The Imitation of Christ*. Beauvoir makes her first communion in tulle and a veil of Irish lace (*not* the ensemble in vogue in 1980s Louisiana, alas for the age). But Meg's and Amy's continual mortification at the plainness of their teen clothes, so like Simone's at their age, was a truth of life and of religion that Beauvoir could not forgive. One day a new girl arrives at her school who is rather better dressed than others: "her bobbed hair, her well-cut jumper and box-pleated skirt, her sporty manner, and her uninhibited voice were obvious signs that she had not been brought up under the influence of Saint Thomas Aquinas." Despite Simone's preference for Jo, it's obvious she is a bit of an Amy; she retains a relatable desire to be beautiful and admired that is charming, a reason why you love her, a forgivable but real flaw in her character. In Beauvoir's novels, each stand-in for herself wanders around Paris and the globe, still wanting new ways to be adored.

The object of Simone's own youthful adoration was her best friend, Zaza, written into her memoirs as narrative foil to her own dreams of rebellion. Together they navigated teen life at their school nicknamed *Le Cours Désir*, where Catholicism was the justification provided for various odd expectations. Zaza's mother, who had eight other children as well, "would have thought it immoral to buy in a shop products that could be made at home: cakes, jams, underwear, dresses, and coats." This was not so much for the sake of thrift – thrift being a virtuous but unnecessary ideal for the young women expected to marry men who owned the means of production – as it was a source of desperately needed occupation: the life of wearing beautiful clothes and sitting up straight at correct social gatherings can only take up so many hours of the day. And so Zaza is sent out to compare the prices of cloth or set to work canning great quantities of jam so that she'll have hardly any time to talk to Simone. (In *The Second Sex* Beauvoir is particularly virulent about the destructive tendencies of making jam.) "Zaza," Beauvoir writes with a certain jealousy, "was too much of a Christian to dream of disobeying her mother." But while Zaza obeyed, she also felt the oddity of what religion was asking, on behalf of religion, all the same: "she couldn't bring herself to believe that by trotting off to shops and tea-parties she was observing faithfully the precepts of the Gospel."

The minor privations of Beauvoir's Paris youth pale beside Alcott's, whose family was not only poor but often poor via the pursuit of otherworldly ideals; during their days as fruitarians, the gossip was that Alcott's father forbade them to grow potatoes, on account of their earthly nature. But there are elements to Alcott's life that could well have struck Beauvoir with envy. Beauvoir's higher education came about because her family could not afford to marry her off with the customary dowry, and so she was sent to school to become a teacher. Her father considered her learning a shameful manifestation of his failure, and told her she read too much. For Alcott, on the other hand, while it was no joke to have as one's father a failed Utopianist, wage-refuser, and sometime *philosophe* who somehow never was able to get his best thoughts onto paper, still her family situation came with certain benefits. Bronson Alcott did take Louisa's education seriously, and her family's connections to the transcendentalist Ralph Waldo Emerson, the abolitionist William Garrison, and the Unitarian minister Theodore Parker meant that radical philosophy, radical politics, and radical religion were a natural part of family life – not something desperately held at bay by frantic parents.

Beauvoir, with her budding social conscience, was vaguely assured by authority figures that the condition of the workers was much better these days. Later, she would insist on seeing for herself, traveling far to witness different social conditions at work; her visits to America involved her in a study of the effects of segregation, which proved to be a major impetus for writing *The Second Sex*. Philosophy, including the political sort, became the medium of revolt by which reality, in all its suffering, could finally be truthfully seen.

For Alcott, by contrast, radical care for the poor – not just helping them out on occasion, but trying to think about what social conditions would end poverty – was the Christianity she knew from early youth. The freedom to experience faith in this way is part of the charm of the March girls' lives, even though

> The main problem with the way religion was taught to Beauvoir was that it formed the truth of one sphere of life but not of the rest.

you can hardly tell from any single word they drop that abolition is on their minds; Beauvoir's freedom to let her politics form an overt part of her published works might well be envied by Alcott in turn. It's fascinating to see how their very similar youthful religious experiences were taken in completely different ways by the people who surrounded them. Alcott writes: "A very strange and solemn feeling came over me as I stood there, with no sound but the rustle of the pines, no one near me, and the sun so glorious, as for me alone. It seemed as if I *felt* God as I never did before, and I prayed in my heart that I might keep that happy sense of nearness all my life." For a Unitarian, this was a perfectly reasonable expression of Christianity. But for Beauvoir, it was trying to communicate something like this and failing to have it taken seriously that finally put an end to her interest in religion.

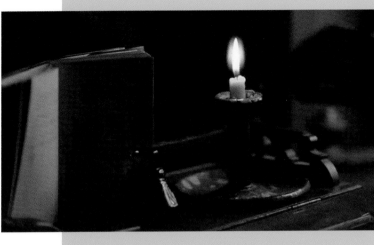

The main problem with the way religion was taught to her, Beauvoir writes, however, was that it formed the truth of one sphere of observable life but not of another: "Sanctity and intelligence belonged to two quite different spheres; and human things – culture, politics, business, manners, and customs – had nothing to do with religion." At first this split was merely puzzling; then Simone smelled a rat. When Pope Leo XIII called for a living wage for workers in *Rerum Novarum* (a moderate position that disavowed anything so threatening as socialism or the abolition of private property), her parents still complained that he "had betrayed his saintly mission," which forced their daughter "to swallow the paradox that the man chosen by God to be His representative on earth had not to concern himself with earthly things."

At university, however, Beauvoir engaged with these ideas via the work of her professor Robert Garric, a "social Catholic" who spoke of providing cultural and intellectual opportunities to the working classes. In him she could admire the co-incidence of idea and life that was missing elsewhere: "At last I had met a man who instead of submitting to fate had chosen for himself a way of life; his existence, which had an aim and a meaning, was the incarnation of an idea, and was governed by its overriding necessity." But she never left behind the taste for the all-or-nothing, her "nostalgia for the Absolute"; as she later famously declared, even socialism was not enough, in her opinion, to bring about women's liberation; the Revolution was needed.

Beauvoir was critical of this aspect of herself, even willing to joke: "a socialist couldn't possibly be a tormented soul; he was pursuing ends that were both secular and limited: such moderation irritated me from the outset. The Communists' extremism attracted me much more; but I suspected them of being just as dogmatic and stereotyped as the

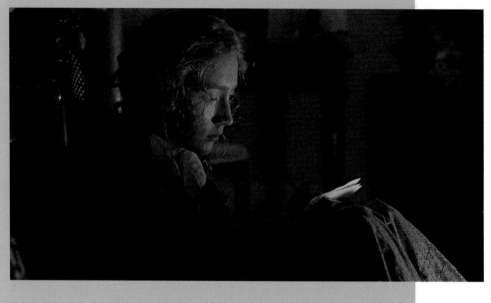

Cathedral School, Sister Hélène, died the year before I would have had her as my teacher. Perhaps enabled by this distance, in 1984 Louisiana was the site of the first successful public prosecution of a priest who sexually abused hundreds of children, in the diocese only a few miles away from mine – a fact that not a single adult mentioned to me, not once, although they did tell me continually to watch out for pedophiles. There was a statue of Saint Vincent de Paul, patron saint of service to the poor, in a little garden outside our church; it was never clear to me just what he was supposed to be famous for.

For our family, Catholicism was a matter of genetics; it certainly wasn't about morality. Certain rules, slightly more complex than those of the other, déclassé denominations, gave a shape to what was allowed and what was not. Everyone lived within and without these rules simply as it happened; if someone needed an annulment, it would be granted eventually, it would just take a while. In Catholic school we learned arguments to defend this complexity from charges of arbitrariness; this somehow formed the totality of theology. It was lacking something, though we knew not what. As Beauvoir puts it, "I had subtle arguments to refute any objection that might be

Jesuits." Beauvoir's 1954 novel *The Mandarins* is a master-class on the fragmentation and foibles of the passionately self-critical left, as its members scrabble to unite themselves after the atrocities of World War II. And her life, devoted to activism not less than to writing, exemplified the co-incidence between word and deed she sought. Crossing the globe to meet with feminist and Marxist activists, writing endless letters in response to readers of *The Second Sex*, she also made her mark at home: Beauvoir's journalism helped tip the balance of French public opinion towards ending the colonial occupation of Algiers.

THE ROMAN CHURCH of Louisiana in the 1980s was and was not the church of Simone's youth. No one asked for mortifications, Rome was far away, and so was France; the last nun at Immaculate Conception

brought against revealed truths; but I didn't know one that proved them."

For me, the problem wasn't so much the proof; epistemology is my least favorite branch of philosophy; it's much more interesting to learn all about things than waste time on how it's possible I know them in the first place. What was missing was more essential. In college I read Martin Luther's *On the Freedom of a Christian* (1520) for the first time. When revelers from the annual campus party interrupted our seminar after a few minutes, I threw my copy against the wall with abandon. I'd never read a text like it; to me at first it seemed like pure absence of thought. But I returned the next morning to the classroom to fish it out of the corner; it wasn't apologetics, but something simpler. The truth, whatever it is, will set you free. I could live with that.

Beauvoir's satisfaction in simple negation of everything religious makes visceral sense to me; I know exactly how it felt because I had to experience it too. To sweep everything away, the artificial constructions, the apparent contempt for the female body and its redemption by self-inflicted wounds, the insistence that human (male) authority was holy *of itself*, that it could always ultimately be trusted: the truth was a prefabricated goal without drama to its completion.

More than this, it wasn't satisfying to be told that there is one season for examining your conscience, as helpful as it is to have a season, with the rest of the year as good as carnival; the power of the confessional takes on a levity in the hands of the youth, a game to play as you get in and out of sin, that's uncomfortable to behold. When I first read Plato I was immediately entranced: here is someone who shows that philosophy is not something to pick up and put down but the only way to really live; someone who hated the love of ignorance as much as I did. Plato, however, notoriously points back up out of the world to a good that permeates it but can't be *of* it – quite.

AFTER ONE NEGATES THE GIVEN, any good Hegelian can tell you, there must come a synthesis which contains *both* the given and its negation in subtler form. Beauvoir, who was otherwise a good Hegelian and knew this well enough, never got there with her negated faith because she didn't want to. She tried to satisfy herself with earthly loves; we love her novels because in them she admits it never worked. In her youth, Beauvoir would go into churches to sit with a quiet moment; I still do the same. But what a relief it is not to be sorry that I can let myself in good faith want the thing the building is supposed to house – the thing that the atheist says, with impossible absolutism, cannot exist, and the thing Aquinas says, too blithely, that all men speak of as God. To be the heir not of the nineteenth century but of Beauvoir's rebellion is unmerited gift; I'll take it.

Beauvoir was happy in college, though she didn't quite find any author from the history of philosophy she felt she could trust; the interpretation of Plato that she was offered seems particularly uninspired, and no one

> Finally, one night, failing to summon God directly then and there, Beauvoir called it quits.

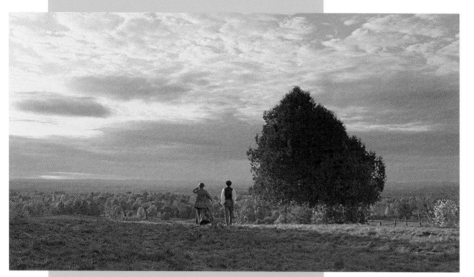

her sense of the importance of art and its promise of longevity, and so at odds with the work of her life.

Her truer feelings are perhaps expressed by this: "If I were describing in words an episode of my life, I felt that it was being rescued from oblivion, that it would interest others, and so be saved from extinction." This sentiment is uncannily echoed in the dialogue of Jo and Amy (as Gerwig renders it in the movie), when they discuss why the writing of a family life of women might have any importance. In the end, Beauvoir as artist and philosopher holds on to this kind of eternity, at least, and with a brilliance that makes me not only full of love but of pride – proud of her and each of the beautiful things she managed to write despite their imperfections, as proud as I am of Alcott for her work and her life, and as proud as we all are of Jo. Not nostalgia but pride, I realized, was my primary feeling when watching Gerwig's film: not in Alcott's perfection, or Gerwig-Jo's aesthetically embalmed autonomy, but that Alcott wrote, and that we read. Beauvoir was not wrong about art.

and no one taught Hegel or Marx at all. She thought literature was a better medium than the "abstract voice" of philosophy, but she struggled with the idea of writing as vanity. In this phase, she grew thoughtful about the possibility of mysticism – she picked up Plotinus and tried to think herself into some direct revelation of the absolute. "In moments of perfect detachment when the universe seems to be reduced to a set of illusions and in which my own ego was abolished, something took their place: something indestructible, eternal; it seemed to me that my indifference was a negative manifestation of a presence which it was perhaps not impossible to get in touch with." She asked her Catholic peers and a teacher if she was on to something. They said no. Her confessor had long ago made it clear he had nothing to say to her doubts.

Finally, one night, failing to summon God directly then and there, she called it quits, concluding, "I should have hated it if what was going on here below had had to end up in eternity." And so her atheism remained on the books. But this remark is at odds with

S HE DID NOT LEARN Jo's lesson, though, or perhaps she learned it too well: she chose a Laurie for a partner after all, or rather a Professor Bhaer (the man Jo did marry) who in her story retains several aspects suspiciously reminiscent of Laurie's worst qualities. That is to say, Beauvoir found Jean-Paul Sartre, and

biography helpfully reminds us, Beauvoir was an existentialist and a philosopher long before Sartre failed his first attempt at the Sorbonne's exam – and then needed her help understanding Leibniz, Husserl, Hegel, and so on – we still see her commitment to what she insists is *his* philosophy, even when describing what was her idea in the first place. When Beauvoir's writing stumbles it's often because it suddenly has a tinge of the apologetics she otherwise despises, that is, when she feels it necessary to apologize for Sartre. That her writing so often successfully breaks free of this, as she in her private life soon broke free of Sartre as partner or idol in truth (after a few months together she declared him a friend of her heart, rather than a subject of lasting adoration), is a testament to the reality of her commitment to freedom as the highest good.

Sartre, in his philosophy, could never quite let go of the willful misreading of Hegel that his youthful self persisted in. It comes down to the dialectical relation between Hegel's master and slave: Sartre took this passage to mean that the human being could never outrun its desire to dominate the Other, of whatever variety: the foreigner, the worker, your lover, the person you pass in the street. Beauvoir wrote *The Ethics of Ambiguity* (1947) in order to defend existentialism against the charge that it lacked a coherent ethics; but her ethical philosophy reached coherence through the understanding that only by willing the freedom of the Other can one reach an authentic understanding and practice of the freedom each individual longs for. This is closer to what Hegel really said. Why was Beauvoir able to listen? She writes: "My Catholic upbringing had taught me never to look on the individual, however lowly, as of no account: everyone had the right to bring to fulfillment what I called their eternal essence." Beauvoir kept what faith she could.

I think Beauvoir settled on atheism because she was unable to imagine an intellectual Christianity. This was not because intellectualism was lacking from the Thomism or Catholic existentialism that she had come across, but because what she wanted was the freedom of a Christian, the freedom to understand God, truth, the Absolute on her own terms, and she was told that there was no way to do this. There's an irony in her captivation with Sartre's vision, which she found novel, of the freedom to will one's own future – all too strangely reminiscent of the argument Luther made in 1520. For Beauvoir, the blind nationalism of the French Catholic church, its triumphal support of colonization, its unwillingness to call private property into question, failed to answer her desire for understanding a world in thrall to capitalism. One must think of Beauvoir as a rebel angel. ❧

> "My Catholic upbringing had taught me never to look on the individual, however lowly, as of no account: everyone had the right to bring to fulfillment what I called their eternal essence."
> Simone de Beauvoir

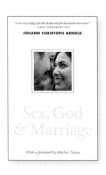

## Sex, God, and Marriage

*Johann Christoph Arnold; Foreword by Mother Teresa*

In this classic book, Arnold, a pastor for over forty years, provides fresh biblical insights into critical issues including the sacredness of sex, the struggle against temptation, the decision to remain single or to marry, child rearing, homosexuality, divorce and remarriage.

**J. I. Packer, Regent College:** Simple and short, but deep, this is one of the best books on handling sexuality in a way that honors God.

**Pope Benedict XVI:** I am very happy for this book and for its moral conviction.

**Softcover, 194 pages, $12.00**

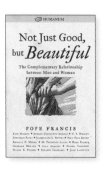

## Not Just Good, but Beautiful

The Complementary Relationship between Man and Woman

*Pope Francis, Rick Warren, N. T. Wright, Gerhard Cardinal Müller, Jonathan Sacks, Wael Farouq, M. Prudence Allen, Nissho Takeuchi, Jean Laffitte, Ignacio Ibarzabal, Kala Acharya, Jacqueline C. Rivers, Tsui Ying Sheng, Henry B. Eyring, and Russell Moore*

Contributors bring the wisdom of their faiths and cultures to bear on this timely issue, examining, celebrating, and illustrating the natural union of man and woman in marriage as a universal cornerstone of healthy families, communities, and societies.

**Softcover, 174 pages, $12.00**

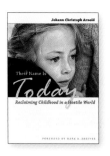

## Their Name Is Today

Reclaiming Childhood in a Hostile World

*Johann Christoph Arnold; Foreword by Mark K. Shriver*

There's hope for childhood. Despite a perfect storm of hostile forces that are robbing children of a healthy childhood, courageous parents and teachers who know what's best for children are turning the tide.

**Jonathan Kozol, author:** Beautiful . . . It is Arnold's reverence for children that I love.

**Publishers Weekly:** A deeply inspiring tribute to children. . . . Arnold's basic message is clear, and well worth heeding.

**Softcover, 189 pages, $14.00**

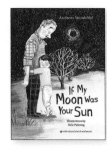

## If My Moon Was Your Sun

*Andreas Steinhöfel; Illustrated by Nele Palmtag; Music by Bizet and Prokofiev*

Did you hear about the boy who kidnapped his grandpa from a nursing home? This delightful tale helps children talk about Alzheimer's and losing a grandparent.

**Nominated for the 2021 Astrid Lindgren Memorial Award**

**School Library Journal, starred review:** With its loving portrayal of aging, caring for the elderly, and the keen nature of kids' sensibilities, this is a must-purchase for all libraries serving children.

**Hardcover, 80 pages, $19.00 with a CD**

**All books 40% off for *Plough Quarterly* subscribers. Use code PQ40 at checkout.**

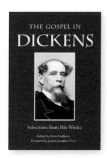

## The Gospel in Dickens
### Selections from His Works

*Edited by Gina Dalfonzo; Foreword by Karen Swallow Prior*

Wish you had time to re-read and enjoy that daunting stack of Charles Dickens novels? Take heart: Dickens enthusiast Gina Dalfonzo has done the heavy lifting for you.

**Gary Colledge, author, *God and Charles Dickens:*** A marvelous glimpse into the mind and soul of Charles Dickens.

**Softcover, 264 pages, $18.00**

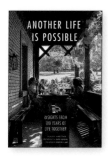

## Another Life Is Possible
### Insights from 100 Years of Life Together

*Created by Clare Stober; Photographs by Danny Burrows; Foreword by Rowan Williams*

This Humans of New York–style book on lived Christian socialism includes profiles of one hundred members of the Bruderhof, past and present, and encompasses themes of technology, education, and sharing everything.

**San Francisco Book Review:** A laudable centennial presentation for this community that also serves to introduce this group to the general public.

**Booklist:** This beautifully produced book, sure to draw in the spiritually curious, is a centenary celebration of the Bruderhof. . . . The accounts all share a sense of having come home, and of finding peace in not having to prove one's worth or achieve material success.

**Hardcover, 320 pages, $40.00**
**anotherlifeispossible.com**

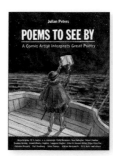

**NEW RELEASES**

## Poems to See By
### A Comic Artist Interprets Great Poetry

*Julian Peters*

A fresh twist on 24 classics, these visual interpretations by comic artist Julian Peters will change the way you see the world.

**Library Journal:** Peters's virtuosity as an illustrator and keen understanding of the texts included here result in a beautiful, memorable volume.

**The Wall Street Journal:** A wide and varied collection, both in visuals and text. . . . reading *Poems To See By* is a stirring experience.

**Gareth Hinds, *The Iliad:*** By turns whimsical, chilling, and profound, Peters has created a wonderful anthology of classic poems new and old.

**Hardcover, 160 pages, $24.00**

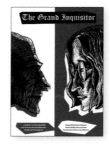

## The Grand Inquisitor
A graphic novel based on the story from Fyodor Dostoyevsky's *The Brothers Karamazov*

*Fyodor Dostoyevsky; Adapted by Natalia Osipova; Illustrated by Elena Avinova; Foreword by Gary Saul Morson*

One of the most famous passages in modern literature, this work raises important questions about free will, human nature, religion, power, and the radically subversive way of Jesus.

**Softcover, 36 pages, $8.00**

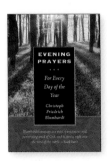
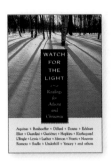
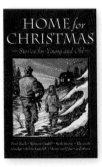
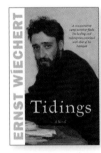

*(continued from page 112)*

he was *all over*"– "Oh, God," she remembers saying aloud, "I did not know you were so *big*." She had a sense too of her own sin. How had she dared to bargain with him? In the words of her biographer, "She began to wish for someone to speak to God for her. . . . At length a friend appeared to stand between herself and an insulted Deity." It was a vision, which "brightened into a form distinct, beaming with the beauty of holiness, and radiant with love." She spoke out loud to it. "I know you, and I don't know you. . . . Who are you?" "Her whole soul," as she described it, "was in one deep prayer. . . . An answer came to her. . . 'It is Jesus.'"

An unexpected answer. She had "heard Jesus mentioned. . . . but had received from what she heard no impression that he was any other than an eminent man, like a Washington or a Lafayette. Now he appeared. . . . And God was no longer a terror and a dread to her."

It was an experience that would remain a guide for the rest of her life.

Shortly afterward, she learned that Dumont had illegally sold her five-year-old son Peter down south to Alabama. She went back to Dumont's house, confronting his wife. "Haven't you as many of 'em left as you can see to?" her former mistress asked. "What have you to support him with, if you could [find him]?" "I have no money," she said, "but God has enough! . . . And I'll have my child again."

"I felt so *tall within*," she said of that moment; "I felt as if the *power of a nation* was with me!" She found Peter, and took the man who had bought him to court. And won: the

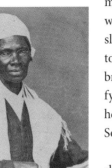

## "I have no money, but God has enough! And I'll have my child again."

Sojourner Truth

first black woman to win a legal battle against a white man in US history.

She was free. And, after July 4 of that year, all of her children were as well. But so many more were not. And where there was not slavery, there was wage slavery. She felt called to travel, to speak about the need for true brotherhood in Christ, "testifying of the hope that was in her." And she took a new name: Sojourner.

Sojourner Truth, 1864

Her travels took her north; she joined an intentional community in Massachusetts, meeting with the lights of the antebellum abolitionist movement: William Lloyd Garrison, Frederick Douglass, and others.

Sojourner Truth lived until 1883, speaking and organizing for abolition and then for women's rights and the abolition of capital punishment. To the end of her days, a fierce personal faith in Christ gave her strength and guided her struggle for a more humane order of society.

She died on November 26, 1883. She is buried with her family in Battle Creek, Michigan.

"I can't read," she explained, in a speech in May of 1851, "but I can hear. I have heard the Bible and have learned that Eve caused man to sin. Well if woman upset the world, do give her a chance to set it right side up again. Jesus. . . . never spurned woman from him. . . . When Lazarus died, Mary and Martha came to him with faith and love and besought him to raise their brother. And Jesus wept – and Lazarus came forth." ⤷

# Sojourner Truth

## SUSANNAH BLACK

### *With Artwork by Jason Landsel*

I N 1844, IN A FIELD outside the town of Northampton, Massachusetts, a gang of young men showed up at a revival meeting, making trouble. The meeting's organizers grew angry; the men – more than a hundred – redoubled their uproar. One of the meeting attendees, a forty-seven-year-old woman, hid behind a chest in the corner of the tent: "I am the only colored person here," she thought, "and on me, probably, their wicked mischief will fall first, and perhaps fatally."

The young men started to rock the tent-poles. And she gave herself a talking-to.

"Shall I run away and hide from the devil? Me, a servant of the living God? Have I not faith enough to go out and quell that mob?" She tried, unsuccessfully, to convince a couple of friends to confront the men with her. She left the tent alone, and, the moon bright on the field, she walked up a rise nearby and began to sing.

Sojourner Truth always was a powerful singer.

It got their attention. And after a few minutes' conversation, she managed to talk them into leaving.

She was born Isabella Baumfree, and grew up in slavery in Rifton, a hamlet in upstate New York. She remembered her mother teaching her the Lord's Prayer in Dutch, her first language. When she was nine, she was sold, along with a flock of sheep, away from her family. At eighteen, she fell in love with Robert, owned by a neighbor of her enslaver, John Dumont; they had a son, James, who died soon after he was born. This relationship didn't sit well with Robert's owner, and she was later made to marry one of Dumont's slaves, Thomas; all their children would then belong to Dumont. She had four more surviving children. Diana was the child of her rape by Dumont; Peter, Elizabeth, and Sophia were her children with Thomas.

S LAVERY IN NEW YORK STATE was on its way out. After July 4, 1827, all enslaved people in the state would be free. After Dumont reneged on a promise to free Isabella a year early, she escaped, taking with her Sophia, who was still a baby. She found a job with a Quaker couple, Mr. and Mrs. Van Wagenen, in nearby New Paltz, New York.

She had had, as she later described it to her biographer Olive Gilbert, the habit of bringing her complaints to God, bargaining her good behavior for his doing what she asked. But at the Van Wagenens', she fell out of the habit of prayer. One day, though, she had the first of a remarkable series of experiences. God, she said, showed her, "on the twinkling of an eye, that

*(continued on preceding page)*

---

**Susannah Black** *is an editor of* Plough *and has written for* First Things, Fare Forward, Front Porch Republic, Mere Orthodoxy, *and* The American Conservative. *She lives in New York City.*
**Jason Landsel** *is the artist for* Plough's *"Forerunners" series, including the painting opposite.*